DIABET 5th edition. MEAL PLANNING MADE EASY 5th Edition

Hope S. Warshaw, MMSc, RD, CDE

.American Diabetes Association.

Director, Book Publishing, Abe Ogden; *Managing Editor,* Rebekah Renshaw; *Acquisitions Editor,* Victor Van Beuren; *Production Manager,* Melissa Sprott; *Composition,* Naylor Design, Inc.; *Copy Editor,* Doris Munson; *Cover Design,* Vis-a-Vis Creative; *Printer,* United Graphics, LLC.

Printed in the United States of America
1 3 5 7 9 10 8 6 4 2

The suggestions and information contained in this publication are generally consistent with the *Standards of Medical Care in Diabetes* and other policies of the American Diabetes Association, but they do not represent the policy or position of the Association or any of its boards or committees. Reasonable steps have been taken to ensure the accuracy of the information presented. However, the American Diabetes Association cannot ensure the safety or efficacy of any product or service described in this publication. Individuals are advised to consult a physician or other appropriate health care professional before undertaking any diet or exercise program or taking any medication referred to in this publication. Professionals must use and apply their own professional judgment, experience, and training and should not rely solely on the information contained in this publication before prescribing any diet, exercise, or medication. The American Diabetes Association—its officers, directors, employees, volunteers, and members—assumes no responsibility or liability for personal or other injury, loss, or damage that may result from the suggestions or information in this publication.

Jane Chiang, MD, conducted the internal review of this book to ensure that it meets American Diabetes Association guidelines.

∞ The paper in this publication meets the requirements of the ANSI Standard Z39.48-1992 (permanence of paper).

American Diabetes Association titles may be purchased for business or promotional use or for special sales. To purchase more than 50 copies of this book at a discount, or for custom editions of this book with your logo, contact the American Diabetes Association at the address below or at booksales@diabetes.org.

American Diabetes Association
1701 North Beauregard Street
Alexandria, Virginia 22311

DOI: 10.2337/9781580405430

Library of Congress Cataloging-in-Publication Data
Warshaw, Hope S., 1954-
Diabetes meal planning made easy / Hope S. Warshaw, MMSc, RD, CDE. -- 5th edition.
pages cm
Includes bibliographical references and index.
ISBN 978-1-58040-543-0 (alk. paper)
1. Diabetes--Diet therapy. I. Title.
RC662.W315 2015
2015014058

To people at risk of and with prediabetes and diabetes:

May the words on the pages ahead motivate, encourage,
and empower you to take actions to eat healthfully.
May eating healthier day after day help you more easily and
successfully manage all aspects of your prediabetes or
diabetes to stay healthier for years to come.

Contents

Introduction to the 5th Edition

By opening **Diabetes Meal Planning Made Easy,** 5th edition, you've signaled that you're ready to take slow and steady steps to eat healthier. I applaud your effort!

Whether you were diagnosed with prediabetes or type 2 diabetes yesterday, had either condition for many years, or just found out you're at high risk for type 2 diabetes, this book can be a vital resource. It will help you uncover the facts about healthy eating—from what to eat to the practical skills of shopping, planning, and preparing healthy meals, as well as tips to eat healthier restaurant meals.

Hands down, putting the knowledge and skills into practice to eat healthy day after day is THE most difficult part of taking care of diabetes, especially in today's fast-paced, convenience-driven world.

Diabetes Meal Planning Made Easy helps you understand the step-wise changes to make in your eating habits and food choices, particularly how to make the changes that give you the biggest bang for your efforts. You'll get to assess your current food and eating habits and pinpoint those that are harming your health. You'll also figure out how to continue to enjoy foods you love to eat, albeit perhaps a bit less of them, less often.

A healthy eating plan is an essential component of your care plan, whether or not you take one or more medications to lower your blood glucose or take other medications to control your blood pressure, lipids (blood fats like LDL cholesterol), and other related or unrelated health conditions.

Keep this statement top of mind: Research shows that the absolute surest way to stay healthy with prediabetes or diabetes is to get and keep your ABCs—blood glucose (A for A1C), blood pressure (B), and lipids (C for cholesterol)—in the target ranges and keep them there over the years. Yes, prediabetes and type 2 diabetes are progressive diseases, but you have the power to slow this progression. Please start to take action NOW!

What you won't find in this book is a one-size-fits-all "diabetic diet" or a magic bullet approach to lose weight and keep it off. Why? It doesn't exist!

You've picked up the right book if you want an approach to healthy living that helps you slowly change your eating habits for the rest of your life, lose weight (if you need to), and keep those lost pounds off for years to come. You'll learn taking these actions can be especially powerful medicine if you act early. Please jump in. There's no time to wait!

Diabetes Meal Planning Made Easy is divided into three sections:

Section 1: Diabetes, Nutrition, and Healthy Eating Basics

Learn about type 2 diabetes and prediabetes along with the latest research and recommendations on healthy eating to manage diabetes. Gather food and nutrient basics. Develop an understanding of the range of healthy eating patterns (ways of eating) you can choose from. Figure out how to personalize YOUR eating plan. Last, gather research-based tips to successfully lose weight and keep those pounds off.

Section 2: Foods by Group

Gain in-depth knowledge about each food group, including starches and grains, fruits, vegetables, milk, yogurt, and protein. Learn about other foods you eat and drink including: fats and oils; sweets, desserts, and sugary foods; alcoholic and non alcoholic beverages; and combination foods like pizza, soups, and frozen meals. Explore easy ways to eat more or less of these foods to achieve your nutrition and diabetes goals.

Section 3: How to Put Healthy Eating into Action

Apply the knowledge and strategies you gained from sections 1 and 2 to plan, shop for, and prepare healthy meals and snacks. Underline the word "plan". Planning is an absolutely essential skill to put into practice for success. Learn how to set short-term goals and evaluate their effectiveness to achieve and maintain the healthy behavior changes you choose to make.

Think of your healthy eating plan, healthier habits, and diabetes management as long-term works in progress. Take one baby step at a time. View any itsy-bitsy change you make towards healthier eating and living as a step in the right direction. Slowly link together lots of tiny tweaks in your lifestyle. Over time you'll build up steam and experience success. Eventually you will have achieved BIG CHANGES.

Don't go gung-ho and try to change everything at once. That's often not a successful long-term solution. And don't beat yourself up if you get off track. Remember: you're human. Learn from the times you veer off track. Then just move forward.

Be mindful that making healthy behavior and lifestyle changes isn't simple or easy. You'll need fortitude, perseverance, and ongoing, frequent support. Find a local or online supportive network of health-care providers, diabetes educators, and people with diabetes to maximize your success.

Success breeds success. You can do this! Good luck!

First, Assess Yourself

Before you turn the page, take a few minutes to create an honest appraisal of your current food choices and eating habits. Create a form like this, or use a form available online. Keep records for a few days. Be honest! No one needs to see this but you. If you're honest, particularly about the amounts of food you eat (you may want to weigh and measure some foods), you'll more easily identify areas for improvement. Once you've got your appraisal, identify a few easy changes to make. Then set a few goals to take action. Over time, repeat this cycle. This is how you start to change your eating habits and lifestyle for good. Read more in chapter 19.

Time	Food	Food Preparation	Amount You Eat

Nutrition and Healthy Eating Basics

CHAPTER 1

About Type 2 Diabetes (and Prediabetes) and Why It Happens

What's Ahead?

➡ Definitions of prediabetes and type 2 diabetes.
➡ Target goals for blood glucose, blood pressure, and lipids (blood fats)—your ABCs—and why they matter.
➡ How prediabetes and type 2 diabetes happen.
➡ Healthy lifestyle actions to help prevent, reverse, or slow down the progression of prediabetes and type 2 diabetes.

Definitions of Prediabetes and Type 2 Diabetes

If you have diabetes (any type), your body has difficulty converting the food you eat into the energy your cells can use to keep your body functioning. After you eat, your body breaks down some foods into glucose (the more scientific and accurate term for "sugar" used in this book). Glucose is the basic fuel for all of the body's cells.

Insulin, a hormone normally produced in sufficient supply by the beta cells of the pancreas, helps move the glucose from your blood into your cells.

When you start to develop prediabetes or type 2 diabetes, several things start to go awry with the fine balance between key hormones responsible for blood glucose control. This process can take years to develop, which is why noticing these conditions early (the earlier the better!) gives you the best shot of reversing or at least slowing down this progression. Learn about the cascade of events that occur on pages 6–8.

Managing diabetes translates to keeping your blood glucose levels as close to normal as much as possible over the years. It's the combination of high blood glucose levels, high blood pressure, and abnormal lipid levels over time that can cause the long-term chronic complications of diabetes.

The most common complications of type 2 diabetes are heart and blood vessel diseases, typically heart attacks and strokes. Another name for these is "macrovascular diseases," which simply means diseases of the body's large blood vessels. They're the leading causes of health problems and death for people with type 2 diabetes. People with many years of type 2 diabetes can also have microvascular complications of the small blood vessels in the eyes, kidneys, and nerves. Enough bad news!

The good news is that if you have prediabetes or are in the early years of type 2 diabetes, if you lose and keep off 5–7% of your weight, you can slow disease progression and dramatically improve the ABCs of diabetes management (see Table 1.1 for goals):

- A = blood glucose and A1C levels. A1C, an abbreviation for hemoglobin A1c or glycated hemoglobin, is an average of all of a person's blood glucose levels over the past 2–3 months. The result is reported as a percentage.

- B = blood pressure.

- C = cholesterol (lipid levels). This includes total cholesterol: low-density lipoprotein cholesterol (LDL cholesterol, the unhealthy type), high-density lipoprotein cholesterol (HDL cholesterol, the healthy type), and triglycerides.

The American Diabetes Association recommends that most people with type 2 diabetes also need to take a blood glucose–lowering medication soon after diagnosis, as well as other medications to keep the ABCs in the target range. To continue to reach these targets over the years, you'll likely need to take additional blood glucose–lowering and other medications. However, and this is important, taking medication doesn't replace healthy eating, being physically active, and managing your weight. These therapies are ALWAYS important elements of your care plan.

How Prediabetes and Type 2 Diabetes Happen

The Centers for Disease Control and Prevention (CDC) estimates that over 86 million Americans have prediabetes. According to recent estimates from the National Institutes of Health, 83% of adults over 65 years old are estimated to have prediabetes!

Prediabetes is defined as the point when blood glucose levels are higher than normal but not high enough to be diagnosed as diabetes (Table 1.2). These numbers keep rising because of the increas-

TABLE 1.1 American Diabetes Association Recommendations for ABC Goals*		
A is for . . . A1C or blood glucose	B is for . . . Blood pressure	C is for . . . Cholesterol or blood lipids
A1C: <7%	<140/90 mmHg	LDL: <100 mg/dL
Fasting and before meals blood glucose: 80–130 mg/dL		HDL: >50 mg/dL women >40 mg/dL men
Blood glucose 1–2 hours after the start of a meal: <180 mg/dL		Triglycerides: <150 mg/dL

*The American Diabetes Association recommends these ABC targets for most people with diabetes; however, there are exceptions. You and your health-care providers should decide which goals are right for you based on your individual situation, age, and health.

ing number of people (including children) who are overweight (defined as up to 30% above normal body weight) or obese (defined as greater than 30% above normal body weight).

But genes also play a role. Not everyone who is overweight or obese develops prediabetes or type 2 diabetes. To develop either condition, you've got to have both insulin resistance and an inability to keep up with your body's demand for insulin (reduced insulin secretion). Genes influence the amount of insulin people can produce. People who inherit genes linked to type 2 diabetes over time may not be able to make enough insulin to overcome their insulin resistance.

Most people with prediabetes don't know they have it. According to the most recent estimates from the CDC, only 11% of the 86 million people estimated to have prediabetes know they have it. Even more, estimates show that not nearly enough people who've been diagnosed take action.

If you suspect you (or a loved one) have prediabetes or type 2 diabetes, take the American Diabetes Association Risk Test: www. diabetes.org/are-you-at-risk/diabetes-risk-test (search "American Diabetes Association risk test"). If the results suggest you may have diabetes, talk to your health-care provider first, and then develop your plan of action if you are at high risk. If you have prediabetes (diagnosed or not) and take no actions to reverse or slow its progression, you may eventually develop type 2 diabetes.

Yes, the time for action IS NOW! Step one? Follow the healthy eating guidelines in this book.

In the last two decades, research has revealed a more complete understanding of how untreated prediabetes commonly progresses into type 2 diabetes. Read the following as you view Fig. 1.1).

Here's what typically happens over time:

- **Excess weight and physical inactivity kickstart the progression.** Excess weight (fat, which is called adipose tissue) causes an increase in and release of substances into the bloodstream, some of which are called cytokines. Cytokines indicate the presence of chronic inflammation, which further fuels the inflammation.

- **Inflammation causes insulin resistance to escalate.** Inflammation doesn't allow the insulin you still make to effectively get glucose into the body's cells.

- **With inflammation and insulin resistance, the body powers up the beta cells to make and put out more insulin.** Larger amounts of insulin are put out into the bloodstream in an attempt to control blood glucose levels. This is typically when blood pressure may start to rise and blood lipids become abnormal.

- **Insulin production from beta cells begins to dwindle.** Blood glucose levels slowly start to rise above normal for the first time. Initially, blood glucose levels after eating tend to run higher than glucose levels after hours of not eating (fasting).

- **Blood pressure rises, lipids become abnormal** (if they haven't already done so). Typically people with this situation have a low HDL, high triglycerides, and unhealthy (but not too elevated) LDL levels, causing an increased risk of cardiovascular disease.

- **Blood glucose climbs slowly.** The beta cells slowly become exhausted and can no longer make enough insulin to keep blood

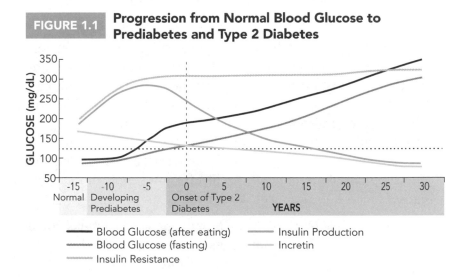

| FIGURE 1.1 | **Progression from Normal Blood Glucose to Prediabetes and Type 2 Diabetes** |

glucose at normal levels. This is when fasting blood glucose levels also rise, and the A1C level rises high enough to diagnose either prediabetes or type 2 diabetes (see Table 1.2). This subtle process can take 5 years or more in adults, but research shows it may happen more quickly in children and adolescents.

- **Over the years with type 2 diabetes, the ability of the pancreas to make a sufficient amount of insulin continues to dwindle, and insulin resistance continues to increase.**

Three Other Hormones Aid Glucose Control

You may think insulin is the only hormone involved with blood glucose control. Not so! The fine balance of blood glucose control is under the influence of three additional hormones. This fine balance is thrown off as prediabetes and type 2 diabetes progress:

- **Amylin,** also made in the beta cells of the pancreas, slows the release of glucose into the bloodstream after eating by slowing stomach emptying and increasing the feeling of fullness. People with type 2 diabetes have a dwindling supply of amylin (an amylin deficiency). An insufficient supply of amylin causes glucose to rise faster after eating.

- **Incretins,** a group of hormones put out from the intestines, including glucagon-like peptide 1 (GLP–1), enhance the pancreas's release of insulin. This in turn slows stomach emptying, promotes fullness, and delays the release of glucose into the bloodstream. It also prevents the pancreas from releasing glucagon, which puts less glucose into the bloodstream. Figure 1.1 on page 7 shows that incretin production wanes with the development of prediabetes. An insufficient supply of incretins causes glucose to rise faster after eating.

- **Glucagon,** made in the alpha cells of the pancreas, breaks down glucose stored in the liver and muscles as glycogen and releases it to provide energy when glucose from food isn't available.

TABLE 1.2 Criteria for the Diagnosis of Prediabetes and Diabetes*	Healthy, No Diabetes	Prediabetes	Diabetes (type 1, 2)
Fasting blood glucose	100 or below	100–125	126 or higher
Random blood glucose	140 or below	140–199	200 or higher
A1C (done in a lab, not a home test)#	5.6% or below	5.7–6.4%	6.5% or higher

Note: If the results from one test are not convincingly indicative of the diagnosis, then a repeat test should be done on a different day.

*Does not apply to pregnant women and gestational diabetes.

#A1C has become the preferred test to diagnose prediabetes and diabetes.

Source: American Diabetes Association, Standards of Medical Care for Diabetes—2016.

Think of glucagon and insulin as hormones with opposite actions. An oversupply of glucagon puts too much glucose into the bloodstream.

Can You Stop, Reverse, or Slow the Progression of Type 2 Diabetes?

The evidence is mounting from large studies conducted around the globe, including China, Finland, and the U.S., that if prediabetes or a high risk of type 2 diabetes is detected early, it can be reversed or slowed. As participants in several of these studies continue to be observed over time, we learn more about the key factors and actions for success.

The most significant predictors of reversing elevated blood glucose levels and attaining normal blood glucose levels with prediabetes are lower blood glucose levels when fasting and after eating, younger age, greater insulin-making capacity, and taking and keeping off weight over the years. Early detection, immediate lifestyle changes, and continuing to practice a healthy lifestyle can be beneficial to your health!

The key point from all of these type 2 diabetes prevention studies is that the optimal way to lose weight—and keep as much of it off as possible—is to make slow and steady changes in your eating habits toward achieving a healthier lifestyle. That's exactly what this book is all about!

While losing weight and keeping it off gets the award for best actor (or actress), these prevention studies show that physical activity earns a supporting role award and is even more important to help you keep weight off. These studies and others underscore the challenge of keeping as many of those lost pounds off as possible. The body simply wants to put those darn pounds on again. (Read more about this in chapter 7.)

The type 2 diabetes prevention studies also show that you need to seek and find support to achieve your goals. Read more about getting the support you need in chapter 23.

Type 2 Diabetes Prevention Studies

The large (~3,000 participants) and lengthy (initially 3-year) study conducted in the U.S. by the National Institutes of Health (NIH) in people at high risk for type 2 diabetes began in the late 1990s and was called the Diabetes Prevention Program (DPP). There were three study groups: intensive lifestyle, standard care with metformin, and standard care (the control group). The intensive lifestyle and standard care with metformin groups were compared to standard care study subjects. Participants in the intensive lifestyle group were encouraged to lose 5–7% of their initial weight, mainly by limiting their calorie and fat consumption, and to exercise for 150 minutes per week. They received regular education and behavioral counseling for 16 weeks initially and less frequently over the 3 years of the DPP. These participants reduced their progression to type 2 diabetes more than the metformin group (see Table 1.3 for statistics). They also had lower blood pressure, had improved blood lipids, and needed fewer medications and lower doses of them to control these conditions.

The Diabetes Prevention Program Outcome Study (DPPOS) is the long-term follow-up study to the DPP and is still ongoing. Results from the study published after 10 years and 15 years are detailed in Table 1.3. The 10-year results, published in 2009, showed that participants lost most of the weight they would lose by about 6 months to 1 year after starting their efforts. It also showed that over time people regain some of the weight they've lost. The DPPOS continues as an observational study, so stay tuned.

Diagnosis of Type 2 Diabetes

You may have been diagnosed with type 2 diabetes just after your blood glucose level crossed the threshold from prediabetes to type 2 diabetes. You may have not even known you had prediabetes. Or it may be a few years before you discover that your blood glucose is high enough for you to be diagnosed with diabetes. You're not alone; millions of people have undiagnosed diabetes. It's more than likely that when you're diagnosed with type 2 diabetes, you are carrying around extra pounds—nearly 80% of people diagnosed with type 2 diabetes are. These factors

TABLE 1.3	DPP/DPPOS Results: Reduction of Incidence of Type 2 Diabetes in a High-Risk Population	
	Intensive Lifestyle	Care with Metformin* Standard
DPP[1]	58%	31%
DPPOS at 10 years[2]	34%	18%
DPPOS at 15 years[3]	27%	17%

*Compared to the standard-care-only study subjects who received no additional education or medication. All DPP participants were offered lifestyle intervention in the DPPOS observational phase of the study, leading to a reduction in differences over time.[3]

1. Diabetes Prevention Program Research Group. Reduction in the incidence of type 2 diabetes with lifestyle intervention or metformin. N Engl J Med 2002;346:393–403.

2. Diabetes Prevention Program Research Group. 10-year follow-up of diabetes incidence and weight loss in the Diabetes Prevention Program Outcomes Study. Lancet 2009;374 (9702):1677–1686.

3. Diabetes Prevention Program Research Group. Long-term effects of lifestyle intervention or metformin on diabetes development and microvascular complications over 15-year follow-up: Diabetes Prevention Program Outcomes Study. Lancet Diabetes Endocrinol. 2015;3:866–875.

and others will influence how you and your health-care provider manage your condition.

The recommendations for how to manage type 2 diabetes have changed dramatically in the last decade and will continue to change. This is due in part to better understanding of the progressive nature of the disease and the availability of more and more medications and advances in diabetes technology. Learn about optimal care, and make sure your providers help you implement a care plan in accordance with the American Diabetes Association's Standards of Medical Care, which are published in January of every year. Research, including that from the Look AHEAD (Action for Health in Diabetes) study (below), shows that early and aggressive actions are the key to slowing down the progression of type 2 diabetes.

The Look AHEAD Study in Type 2 Diabetes

The Look AHEAD study was conducted in the U.S. from the early 2000s to 2012. It was funded by NIH. Look AHEAD is the largest and longest (to date) randomized, clinical study focusing on the use of an intensive lifestyle program (similar to the one used in the DPP) to promote weight loss in overweight people with relatively early-onset type 2 diabetes (they were diagnosed from 3 months to 13 years before entering the study). The study had an intensive lifestyle group and a control group that received standard care. The main focus was to answer the question of whether weight loss and maintenance of that lost weight, along with physical activity early in the disease, could help prevent or delay heart and blood vessel problems usually associated with type 2 diabetes.

Interestingly, the same pattern of weight loss as in the DPP/DPPOS was seen (see Table 1.3). Maximum weight loss occurred in the first 6 months to a year, then a slow and steady climb back to, but still below, starting weight. (This is a very typical observation in weight loss studies.) The same was true for A1C. Participants lowered their A1C the most in the first year, and it slowly crept back up but remained lower in the intensive lifestyle group versus the control group at the end of the study.

This study was stopped 2 years early because it did not show that weight loss in the intensively treated group sufficiently lowered the incidence of heart and blood vessel diseases (heart attacks and strokes) to warrant continuing the study. A number of factors for these results were cited by the researchers: a healthier-than-average study population, improved care after heart attacks or strokes, and improved control of risk factors (for example, many participants took statin medications to lower their LDL cholesterol).

However, there were many other health and quality-of-life benefits realized by the intensive lifestyle participants:

- Less and fewer blood glucose–lowering, blood pressure, and lipid-improving medications taken as participants generally achieved improved ABCs (with fewer medications).

- Lower incidence of chronic kidney disease.

- Less depression.

- Less sleep apnea (86% of participants had sleep apnea when the study started).

- Less urinary incontinence.

- Reduced self-reported symptoms of diabetes eye disease (retinopathy).

- Less use of health-care resources, a benefit for participants and society at large.

The Look AHEAD study, which continues today as an observational study, is one more study to reinforce the importance of detecting type 2 diabetes as early as possible (better yet, at the prediabetes stage) and to manage it as aggressively as possible over the years to achieve those ABC targets and improve health and quality of life.

If or When You Need Blood Glucose–Lowering Medications

At this point, the U.S. Food and Drug Administration (FDA) has not approved any blood glucose–lowering medication for prediabetes. Several blood glucose–lowering medications have been tested and used in diabetes prevention studies, including metformin. Several of these medications are becoming more widely prescribed for prediabetes. Health-care providers prescribe them "off label." (Medication use is considered "off label" when the medication is not being prescribed for its FDA-approved use.) Metformin is an insulin sensitizer, which means it treats insulin resistance by preventing the liver from overproducing glucose. It also helps the muscles use excess glucose. Metformin is generic, low cost, and has been well studied for many years. There's also evidence that it may lower the risk for heart disease and some weight-related cancers.

Unfortunately, by the time a person is diagnosed with type 2 diabetes, it's estimated that they have already lost between 50 and 80% of their beta cell function. This is the reason that the American Diabetes Association and other expert groups recommend that most people with type 2 diabetes start on at least one blood glucose–lowering medication at the time of diagnosis, typically metformin (unless there's a reason a person can't take it).

If blood glucose levels at diagnosis are higher than what a healthy lifestyle and metformin may be able to control, a person may need additional blood glucose–lowering medications as well. The need for these may be temporary or permanent based on the person's ability to control blood glucose and manage their weight and lifestyle over time.

To keep blood glucose levels in target ranges over the years and slow the progression of the disease, people usually need to increase the doses of or add other blood glucose–lowering medications to their care plan. The good news today is that there are more and more effective blood glucose–lowering medications and more on the way.

Eventually, many people who live long enough with type 2 diabetes will need to take insulin by injection because their ability to make enough insulin dwindles over the years. If your provider recommends starting insulin, don't hesitate. With thinner, sharper needles; convenient pens, patches, and pumps; and newer insulins, taking insulin has become easier than ever before and will likely get easier over time as newer forms of inhaled insulin are developed. A diabetes educator can be a great supporter as you explore your options and make this transition to insulin. Seek them out!

Your Diabetes Care Plan

Regardless of which medications you use over the years to control your ABCs, good control is hard to achieve without three other elements:

- Healthy eating to get to and stay at a healthy weight.

- Weight loss, with the goal to keep as much lost weight off as possible.

- Getting and staying physically active with three types of activity:
  —**Moderate-intensity aerobic physical activity:** a minimum of 150 total minutes each week at 50–70% of maximum heart rate spread out over at least 3 days per week, with no more than 2 consecutive days without exercise
  —**Resistance training:** two times a week
  —**Less sedentary behavior:** reduction of the amount of time you spend being sedentary (no more than 90 minutes at a time other than when you sleep).

A final note. Whether you have prediabetes or type 2 diabetes, and regardless of what you've done (or not done) in the past, think of today as the first day to take charge. Don't beat yourself up for what you haven't done to this point. And try not to get caught in that denial trap. It's so easy to do so because you typically feel no physical pain with prediabetes or type 2 diabetes. In other words, it's easy to deny you have it or that it's causing any problems, but diabetes can affect your whole body. Start to take action NOW! All of your body parts will thank you in the years to come.

How to Eat Healthy with Diabetes

What's Ahead?

➡ Brief recap of diabetes nutrition recommendations.
➡ Key principles of healthy eating with diabetes.
➡ How the diabetes nutrition recommendations dovetail with the general guidelines for healthy eating.
➡ Eating patterns and those that promote health for people with prediabetes or diabetes.

Brief Recap of Diabetes Nutrition Recommendations

To say the nutrition recommendations for diabetes have changed dramatically over the years is an understatement, and that's not even going back to before 1921 (the pre-insulin days). A review of the last couple of decades uncovers a major revolution. For starters, the phrase "a diabetic diet" is now outdated; no such thing exists.

Next, sugary foods and sweets don't need to be forbidden. There are no forbidden foods! Of course there are foods, mainly due to their undesirable nutrition profiles, whether loaded with added sugars (carbohydrates with no nutrition) or unhealthy fats, that should be on your only-once-in-a-while list.

The American Diabetes Association revises its nutrition recommendations every few years. The revisions include an in-depth review of the research along with discussion and debate among leading experts in the field. You'll find the most recent version of the American Diabetes Association nutrition recommendations for adults at http://professional.diabetes.org/admin/UserFiles/0%20 -%20Sean/dc132042%20FINAL.pdf.

There is no one "diabetic diet" and no one type of eating pattern that "works" best for everyone. Plus, there's no one set number of calories or amounts of foods or nutrients (the calorie-containing ones: carbohydrate, protein, and fat) that is right for everyone. There are fewer "food rules" today than ever before. What is essential is that you and your providers explore a few eating patterns and zero in on one that helps you accomplish your diabetes and nutrition goals over time.

Your providers should be willing to work with you collaboratively. This means you both share your goals for developing an individualized eating plan and approach to managing your diabetes. Your goals need to be realistic and achievable within the context of YOUR life. They need to consider your individual characteristics, preferences, life schedule, and more. Regular and ongoing support is essential to promote healthy behavior changes, control of your ABCs, and your weight. Read more in chapter 23.

Same Song, Different Verse

If you also have heart disease, do you wonder whether there are different eating guidelines to manage that condition? What about eating to manage high blood pressure? Great questions! Get ready for good news. Today, due to lots of health and nutrition research done over the last few decades, there's pretty complete and straightforward advice about foods (and nutrients) to eat more of, and less of, to prevent or control diabetes, heart disease, and high blood pressure. People with type 2 diabetes or at risk of developing diabetes often also have high blood pressure or heart disease. In essence, the healthy eating plans detailed in this book can help you prevent or manage all three health conditions.

The healthy eating guidelines in this book reflect today's American Diabetes Association nutrition recommendations, which echo the 2015–2020 Dietary Guidelines from the federal government (read more about these below). They also mirror the healthy eating guidelines from the American Heart Association and the American Cancer Society. In fact, the American Diabetes Association collaborates with these two important health organizations on an initiative called the Preventive Health Partnership. The Everyday Choices program (www.everydaychoices.org) was created as part of this partnership to communicate the message that healthful eating and living a healthy lifestyle can reduce the risk of and help you manage some cancers, heart and circulatory diseases, prediabetes, and type 2 diabetes.

Diabetes Recommendations and the 2015–2020 U.S. Dietary Guidelines

Federal law requires that the Dietary Guidelines for Americans be reviewed and revised every 5 years by a committee of nutrition and health experts who are appointed by the secretaries of Health and Human Services (HHS) and the U.S. Department of Agriculture (USDA). These guidelines provide the general public with guidance on healthy eating to prevent chronic diseases, like prediabetes and type 2 diabetes. You can read the 2015–2020 Dietary Guidelines at health.gov/dietaryguidelines/2015/guidelines/.

The most recent Dietary Guidelines focused on 10 key healthy eating messages (Table 2.1). As you read through these, observe how closely these guidelines echo the American Diabetes Association nutrition recommendations.

TABLE 2.1 Goals for Healthy Eating

Goal	Dietary Guideline (DG) compared to American Diabetes Association Recommendation (ADA)
1. Calories/weight control	*DG:* Start a healthy eating pattern that accounts for all foods and beverages within an appropriate calorie level.
	ADA: Reduce calorie intake while maintaining a healthful eating plan.
	Translation: To lose weight, eat fewer calories than your body uses. To keep lost weight off, be constantly vigilant about calorie intake and get near-daily physical activity (at least 30 minutes).
2. Sodium	*DG:* Consume less than 2,300 milligrams (mg) per day of sodium.
	ADA: Less than 2,300 milligrams (mg), same as the general population. Further reduction in sodium for people with high blood pressure should be individualized.
	Translation: Consume no more than 2,300 milligrams of sodium each day. This is a tough challenge, but it can be done by eating few processed foods and by eating restaurant foods that are naturally low in sodium. Processed foods are those that have sodium-containing ingredients added in as they are canned, frozen, cured, or otherwise processed before they're sold. Processed foods and restaurant foods contribute about three-quarters of the sodium Americans eat. Several foods, like breads, cold cuts, pizza, poultry, and sandwiches, aren't necessarily high in sodium but, because we eat them so often, contribute a lot of sodium. Salt, which contains sodium, adds about 10% of the sodium we eat. Use as little as you can.
3. Solid fats (saturated and trans fat)	*DG:* Reduce the intake of calories from solid fats. Consume less than 10% of calories from saturated fat by replacing them with healthier monounsaturated and polyunsaturated fats. Keep trans fat consumption as low as possible by limiting foods that contain synthetic sources of trans fats, such as partially hydrogenated oils, and by limiting other solid fats. Use oils to replace solid fats where possible.

continued

TABLE 2.1 *continued*	
Goal	**Dietary Guideline (DG) compared to American Diabetes Association Recommendation (ADA)**
3. Solid fats, (saturated and trans fats), *cont.*	*ADA:* Same as the general population
	Translation: The focus today is less on limiting total fat consumption and more on choosing healthier fats and oils, such as those from vegetables, nuts, or seeds that are mainly monounsaturated and polyunsaturated. Eat 20 to 35% of your calories as fat. Limit foods with saturated and trans fats as much as possible.
4. Added sugars	*DG:* Conume less than 10% of calories/day from added sugars.
	ADA: While substituting sucrose-containing foods for isocaloric [the same] amounts of other carbohydrates may have similar blood glucose effects, consumption should be minimized to avoid displacing nutrient-dense food choices. Limit or avoid sugar-sweetened beverages from any caloric sweetener, including high fructose corn syrup, to reduce weight gain and worsening of heart disease risk factors.
	Translation: Added sugars encompass an array of calorie-containing sweeteners, including high fructose corn syrup, which are added to foods and beverages to sweeten them. All sources of added sugars, including sugar, high fructose corn syrup, brown sugar, maple syrup, and honey, provide a concentrated source of calories and carbohydrates with next to no nutrition. Limit them as much as possible.
5. Whole grains	*DG:* Limit the consumption of foods that contain refined grains, especially refined grain foods that contain solid fats, added sugars, and sodium. Consume at least half of all grains as whole grains. Increase whole-grain intake by replacing refined grains with whole grains.
	ADA: For good health, carbohydrate intake from whole grains is advised.
	Translation: Eat more whole grains and foods that contain whole-grain ingredients, like bread, crackers, and pasta, rather than those made with refined grains. Limit grain-based foods that also contain solid fats, added sugars, or sodium, such as refined grain–based pastries and desserts and crunchy snack foods.

continued

TABLE 2.1 *continued*	
Goal	**Dietary Guideline (DG) compared to American Diabetes Association Recommendation (ADA)**
6. Vegetables and fruits	*DG:* Eat a variety of vegetables, especially dark-green, red, and orange vegetables and legumes (beans and peas).
	ADA: For good health, carbohydrate intake from vegetables and fruits is advised.
	Translation: Eat fruit and vegetables every day. All fruits and vegetables prepared with no or limited added fats and sugars are excellent sources of nutrition.
7. Dairy foods	*DG:* Consume fat-free or low-fat dairy, including milk, yogurt, cheese, or fortified soy beverages.
	ADA: For good health, carbohydrate intake from dairy foods is advised.
	Translation: Americans, including children and young adults, drink, on average, only about one serving of milk a day, when we need at least two 8-ounce servings per day. Fat-free milk is the optimal source of calcium, vitamin D, and other important nutrients.
8. Protein foods	*DG:* Eat a variety of protein foods, including seafood, lean meats and poultry, eggs, beans and peas (legumes), nuts, seeds, and soy products.
	ADA: Evidence is inconclusive for an ideal amount of protein. The amount should be individualized.
	Translation: Choose lean meats, prepare them with limited fat, and enjoy no more than 3–4 ounces cooked meat no more than a couple of times a day. Take the skin off poultry before or after cooking. Enjoy seafood prepared using low-fat methods. Use other healthy non-animal based sources of protein, like legumes (beans and peas), nuts, seeds, and soy-based foods.
9. Alcohol	*DG:* If alcohol is consumed, it should be consumed in moderation—up to one drink per day for women and two drinks per day for men—and only by adults of legal drinking age.
	ADA: Same as for the general population.
	Translation: Practice moderation. The calories add up quickly. Moderate alcohol intake has minimal short- or

continued

TABLE 2.1 *continued*	
Goal	Dietary Guideline (DG) compared to American Diabetes Association Recommendation (ADA)
9. Alcohol, *cont.*	long-term effects on blood glucose levels. Don't drink in excess due to added calories, potential impact on blood glucose control, and potential harm to yourself and others.

Sources: Dietary Guidelines for Americans, 2015-2020. Access www.health.gov/dietaryguidelines/dga2010/DietaryGuidelines2010.pdf.

Evert A, Boucher J, et al. Nutrition therapy recommendations for the management of adults with diabetes. *Diabetes Care* 2013;36(11):3821–3842.

Discover an Eating Pattern Right for You

The term "eating pattern" simply means a combination of foods or food groups shown to promote health and prevent disease. Simply put, it is a way—or your way—of eating. We all have our own way of eating. We don't eat single nutrients, like carbohydrate. We eat foods, like a slice of bread or a piece of chicken, that are packages of nutrients that contain varying amounts and combinations of carbohydrate, protein, and fat. And, due to the combination of nutrients in our foods and the way we tend to eat, there's only so much wiggle room, particularly if you want to eat healthfully, to eat more carbohydrate and less protein and fat, or vice versa.

Is there a best eating pattern for diabetes? No! Research shows that there's a variety of eating patterns that can help people with prediabetes or type 2 diabetes eat healthfully and at the same time achieve their ABC goals.

Several eating patterns were reviewed in the most recent American Diabetes Association nutrition recommendations, including vegetarian, Mediterranean style, lower fat and higher carbohydrate, lower carbohydrate and higher fat, and the DASH (Dietary Approaches to Stop Hypertension) eating plan (developed for the National Institutes of Health's DASH study of people with high blood pressure). (Read more about DASH in chapter 4.)

There's a lot of research out there on eating patterns, and many of those studies involve people with diabetes. But, as researchers love to say, "More research is needed!" What is clear, though, is that there is no one right way to control your weight and ABCs. The RIGHT eating pattern for YOU is one that you can follow now and in the future—one that fits your needs and lifestyle.

What and how much you eat is hardly the only lifestyle factor you can modify to get and stay healthy. Study after study shows that other health behaviors such as being physically active, minimizing sedentary behavior (hours of sitting), not smoking, getting adequate quality and quantity of sleep at the right time of day, and limiting stress are ALL key features of a healthy lifestyle and maintaining a healthy weight.

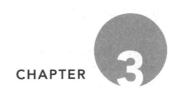

About Calories, Carbohydrate, Protein, and Fat

Calories Defined

Foods supply energy in the form of calories, which are units of energy. The body uses calories to function (to do its work). The body's need for calories, or energy, never stops, even when you sleep. The calories you need each day depend on multiple factors, such as your sex, height, body size, current weight, and whether you've gained or lost weight in the past. (Yes, losing weight can cause your body to need fewer calories at a lower weight. Learn more in chapter 7.) The amount of physical activity you get (or don't) is another significant factor.

Calories are in foods and some beverages. Foods and calorie-containing beverages contain varying amounts of the three nutrients: carbohydrate, protein, and fat. Some foods and beverages contain calories from all three. For example, low-fat (2%) milk contains carbohydrate, protein, and fat, while fat-free milk contains no fat. Fruits contain mainly carbohydrate, a bit of protein, and no fat to speak of. Protein foods like a piece of broiled chicken or fish contain mainly protein and small amounts of fat. In section 2, you'll learn about how much carbohydrate, protein, and fat are in foods and beverages in each food group.

To make use of the calories and nutrients you eat, the body breaks down nutrients through digestion. The body's primary and preferred source of energy is glucose, which comes from the breakdown of foods containing carbohydrate. Glucose can also be created from protein, if needed. For the cells in your body to use the glucose, insulin (whether from the pancreas or via injection or another device, like a patch or pump) is needed to move the glucose into the cells. For people without diabetes, this is a no-brainer. No thinking required! For people with prediabetes or type 2 diabetes, the common problem of insulin resistance can make effective use of the glucose from food a hurdle. In addition, most people with type 2 diabetes also have a relative shortage of insulin being made by and put out from their pancreases. The variety of blood glucose–lowering medications available today, including insulin, can (along with healthy eating) help you use your calories for energy and keep your blood glucose under control.

A fourth source of calories, for people who choose to drink it, is alcohol. Learn all about alcohol and diabetes in chapter 16.

Foods are essentially packages of nutrients that include various mixes of carbohydrate, protein, and fat. How much carbohydrate, protein, and fat you eat is directly related to which foods you eat. For example, if you choose to eat more protein foods than fruits and starches, you'll eat more protein and fat and less carbohydrate just by virtue of the nutrients in those foods. Conversely, if you eat more carbohydrate-rich foods, you'll eat more carbohydrate and less protein and fat. Your goal is to slowly make some changes and zero in on a balance of these nutrients that form your healthy eating plan to help you achieve your goals.

Carbohydrate

Carbohydrates are your body's primary and preferred source of energy because they're easy for the body to break down and get into your cells. There are three types of carbohydrate in foods: starches, fibers, and sugars. Carbohydrates generally contain 4 calories of energy per gram.

Major Carbohydrate Sources

The majority of calories in these foods come from carbohydrate:

- Starches, such as breads, cereals, pasta, and starchy vegetables (such as corn, squash, sweet potatoes, and white potatoes).

- Legumes (beans and peas) (these foods contain most of their calories from carbohydrates, but they do contain more protein per serving than other starches).

- Sugary foods, such as regularly sweetened soda, jellybeans, hard candies, and syrups.

- Sweets, such as desserts, ice cream, cookies, and chocolate bars (though many of the calories in these foods come from fats).

- Vegetables (nonstarchy), such as lettuce, broccoli, and carrots.

- Fruits, such as apples, oranges, fruit juices, and raisins.

- Dairy foods, such as milk and yogurt (cheese contains just a small amount of carbohydrate and mainly protein and fat).

SUGARS, SUGARY FOODS, AND SWEETS

Sugars, sugary foods, and sweets are no longer off-limits for people with diabetes. Fit sugary foods and sweets into your eating plan in small quantities. Remember that sweets are concentrated sources of carbohydrate and calories that can raise blood glucose levels when there is not enough insulin available. Plus, many sweets, such as cheesecake and ice cream, contain a good bit of fat, which usually adds calories and some unhealthy saturated fat. Sweets often offer little in the way of nutrition. Read more about sweets in chapter 14.

DIETARY FIBERS

Most Americans don't eat nearly the recommended amount of fiber (Table 3.1). Research shows less than 4% of Americans meet the recommended goal! Dietary fiber includes the portion of plant-based foods that is not digested plus other functional fibers with health benefits. Our foods contain hundreds of different types of fibers that have different functions and benefits. Some fibers help with digestion and regularity, others improve blood fats (lipids), and others can help with weight control. To stay healthy, you need all types of fibers. Get the variety of fibers you need by eating adequate amounts of whole grains, legumes (beans and peas), fruits, and vegetables (Table 3.2). Learn more about fiber intake in section 2.

Carbohydrate and Diabetes

According to the American Diabetes Association nutrition recommendations, the balance between the amount of carbohydrate you

TABLE 3.1 Recommended Daily Fiber Intake	
Sex and Age (grams/day)	Amount
Men, age 50 and younger	38
Men, age 50 and older	30
Women, age 50 and younger	25
Women, age 50 and older	21

TABLE 3.2	Fibers: Top 10 Food Sources			
Food	Serving	Food Group	Amount (g)	%DV
Bran cereal (e.g., All-Bran, 100% Bran, Fiber One)	1/2 cup	Starch	10–18	40–72
Acorn or butternut squash, cooked	1 cup	Starch	6–9	24–36
Dried peas, beans, and lentils	1/2 cup	Starch	5–8	20–32
Bran flakes	3/4 cup	Starch	4–6	16–24
Raspberries	1 cup	Fruit	8	32
Blueberries	3/4 cup	Fruit	4	16
Brussels sprouts, cooked	1/2 cup	Vegetable	4	
Corn, cooked	1/2 cup	Starch	6	24
Broccoli, spinach, or other greens, cooked	1/2 cup	Vegetable	3	12
Apricots, dried	8 halves	Fruit	3	12

Daily Value = 25 g
Excellent Source = 5 g
Good Source = 2.5–4.75 g

eat and the amount of available insulin your body has when it's needed has the most influence on blood glucose levels after you eat. It's not the amount of carbohydrate you eat alone. If the body has sufficient insulin around when you eat carbohydrates, your body can control blood glucose. Thus, a big goal of blood glucose control is having adequate insulin when it's needed.

Once the carbohydrate in food is broken down to glucose and is in your blood, your cells don't know whether that glucose came from a bunch of jelly beans or a piece of fruit. But your body will! A piece of fruit offers fiber, vitamins, and minerals, whereas jelly beans offer calories with no nutrition. The amount of carbohydrate you eat, not the type of carbohydrate, has the greater effect on your blood glucose level.

Once you learn about how carbohydrate affects blood glucose, it may seem logical to strictly limit the amount of carbohydrate you eat to control your blood glucose. Research has not shown there to be an ideal amount of carbohydrate for people with diabetes, including people with prediabetes or type 2 diabetes who want to lose weight. The bulk of studies show that strictly limiting the amount of carbohydrate you eat, say to 40% or less, may help you lower your blood glucose and help with weight loss initially, but over time it won't likely help you achieve your weight and glucose goals.

To get the fibers, vitamins, and minerals you need for good health, it's important to eat a sufficient amount of carbohydrate from vegetables, fruits, whole grains, legumes, and dairy foods. Getting less than 40% of your calories from carbohydrate, especially if you need to limit your calories per day to around 1,500 calories or less, makes it very difficult to eat sufficient amounts of the fibers, vitamins, and minerals you need.

Limit sources of carbohydrate like refined grains, sugary foods, and sweets, which contain added fats, sugars, and sodium, because they don't offer much nutrition. Quality versus quantity should be a BIG factor in your food choices.

If you're eating healthy amounts and sources of carbohydrate (Table 3.3) and you're not able to control your blood glucose levels, then it's likely you need to work with your health-care providers to start on a blood glucose–lowering medication, increase a medication dose, or add another medication. Remember, as you learned in chapter 1, type 2 diabetes is progressive and most often requires an increasing amount of blood glucose–lowering medications to control it over time.

TABLE 3.3	Recommended Ranges of Carbohydrate, Protein, and Fat for Americans
Macronutrient Name	Range for Percentage of Total Calories
Carbohydrate	45–65%
Protein	10–35%
Fat	20–35%

These recommendations are for adults over 19 years old and don't include women who are pregnant or breast-feeding.

Source: Dietary Reference Intakes for Macronutrients, United States Department of Agriculture. Available from www.nal.usda.gov/fnic/DRI/DRI_Tables/macronutrients.pdf. Accessed 15 October 2015.

Glycemic Index, Glycemic Load, and Blood Glucose

The potential value of applying the concepts of the glycemic index (GI) and glycemic load (GL) in diabetes meal planning has long been the subject of debate. Today, the American Diabetes Association nutrition recommendations suggest that substituting low GI foods for higher GI foods may modestly improve blood glucose control. It's much more important to focus on the total amount of carbohydrate you eat, making sure the sources of carbohydrate you eat are healthy and making sure you have adequate insulin to control blood glucose levels.

Many factors beyond GI contribute to how a food may impact blood glucose levels:

- Blood glucose level at the time you eat.
- Available insulin.
- How much blood glucose–lowering medicine you take, when you take it, and when you eat.
- Level of insulin resistance in general and when you eat the food(s).
- Individual responses to foods and different responses on different days.
- The amount of fiber and whole grains in a meal (these can slow the rise of blood glucose).
- How ripe a fruit or vegetable is .
- Form of the food (for example, fettuccine can affect blood glucose differently than macaroni).
- Variety of the food (for example, long-grain or short-grain rice, Yukon gold or red potatoes, and when and where a product was grown).
- Whether you eat the food raw or cooked (the more a food is cooked, the more likely it is to raise blood glucose quickly).
- The other foods you eat at the time (a meal that is mainly carbohydrate with a small amount of fat may raise your blood glucose more quickly and to a greater degree than a meal with more fat).

Protein

Protein is another source of calories. But unlike carbohydrates, protein isn't your body's preferred source of energy. Proteins are chains of different sequences of amino acids, which are the building blocks of protein. Once you eat protein, the body breaks it down into different sequences of amino acids. The body then uses the amino acids to build a wide variety of different proteins to build, repair, and maintain the body's tissues and help the body function. Hormones like insulin are protein-specific sequences of amino acids. This is the key reason you can't take insulin as a pill. It would be digested like any other protein and no longer would look like insulin to the body!

Protein contains 4 calories of energy per gram (the same as carbohydrate). In this book we'll refer to the foods that mainly contain protein as protein foods. Generally, protein foods are packages of protein and varying amounts of fat. A few, such as fat-free dairy foods and legumes, contain carbohydrate and protein.

Protein Sources

These foods contain most of their calories from protein:
- Red meats (beef, lamb, pork, and veal).
- Poultry (chicken, turkey).
- Seafood, fish, and shellfish.
- Cheese.
- Eggs.

These foods contain moderate amounts of calories from protein:
- Dairy foods, such as milk and yogurt.
- Legumes (beans and peas) (see also the carbohydrates list).
- Nuts (also contain fat).

These foods contain small amounts of calories from protein:
- Starches, such as breads, cereals, pasta, and starchy vegetables.
- Nonstarchy vegetables, such as lettuce, broccoli, and carrots.

Protein and Diabetes

The American Diabetes Association's nutrition recommendations do not suggest an ideal amount of protein for people with diabetes to achieve their ABC goals. The amount you eat should be individualized based on your needs, your goals, and the way you like to eat. However, the amount should be within the Dietary Guidelines of between 10 and 35% of calories. This is not a lot of protein, as you can see in the model meals on pages 67–69. It certainly doesn't allow for an 8-ounce piece of beef, fish, or chicken once or twice a day.

Eating smaller amounts (about 2–4 ounces, cooked) of protein, leaner portions of animal protein, and more non-animal sources of protein can help reduce your intake of saturated and trans fats. Remember that balance, and review Table 3.3. If you choose to eat more protein and fat, you'll likely eat less carbohydrate.

In people with type 2 diabetes, research shows that protein increases the amount of insulin produced by the pancreas (the insulin you still make), but it doesn't increase blood glucose levels. For this reason, there's no need to treat low blood glucose levels (if you experience them) with foods or combinations of foods that contain carbohydrate and protein. Meals that are high in protein and fat (think prime rib with a baked potato loaded with butter and sour cream) have the potential to cause a delayed rise in blood glucose. Checking your blood glucose levels can help you learn how your body reacts to foods like these.

Fat

Fat is the third main source of calories from foods. Fat isn't your body's preferred source of energy, but if the body doesn't have enough calories from carbohydrate or is unable to use the energy from carbohydrate or protein due to an absolute absence of insulin, fat from stored sources can be broken down into what are known as ketones or ketone bodies. Ketones can supply the brain with energy. Ketones are only produced if someone eats nearly no carbohydrate and minimal calories (this condition is known as starvation ketosis) or if someone (usually) with type 1 diabetes goes for a while without enough insulin and has very high blood glucose levels. The resulting condition is called diabetic ketoacidosis (DKA) and is considered a life-threatening emergency.

The fat in foods provides a concentrated source of calories at 9 per gram. That's more than double the calories per gram for carbohydrate and protein. Fat-containing foods have varying amounts of four different fats: saturated, trans, polyunsaturated (including both omega-3 fats and omega-6 fats), and monounsaturated fats. Learn more in chapter 13.

Some of the fat you eat is in the food itself, like the fat in meat, chicken, and cheese. Some is added to foods, such as margarine or butter on a potato, cream cheese on a bagel, and dressing on a salad. Fat is also used when preparing some foods.

Fat Sources

These foods contain nearly all their calories from fat:
- Oils (all types).
- Margarine, butter, and cream cheese.
- Salad dressings, mayonnaise, and sour cream.

These foods contain many calories from fat and some from protein:
- Nuts and seeds.
- Sausage and bacon (regular).

These foods contain varying amounts of calories from fat, depending on several factors, like the cut of meat, whether the poultry is eaten with skin on or off, and whether the food is regular, low-fat, or fat-free:
- Red meats (beef, lamb, pork, and veal).
- Poultry.
- Seafood, fish, and shellfish.
- Cheese.

- Eggs.
- Milk and yogurt.

Fat and Diabetes

It's common for people with prediabetes or type 2 diabetes to have abnormal blood lipid levels (typically unhealthy LDL, low HDL, or high triglycerides) and have or be at increased risk of heart and blood vessel diseases, known generally as macrovascular disease. To minimize problems with heart and blood vessel diseases, control the B and C of your ABCs—that's blood pressure and cholesterol (lipid levels).

The current American Diabetes Association nutrition recommendations do not recommend an ideal amount of fat to eat and suggest that this goal be individualized. In years past, there was more emphasis on eating less total fat, but today the Dietary Guidelines recommend the range of 20–35% of calories from fat (see Table 3.3 [above]). The focus is now squarely on the quality or healthiness of the fats you eat rather than the amounts. However, because fat is a concentrated source of calories, if you are trying to eat fewer calories, it will be important to carefully monitor how many grams of fat you eat as well as choosing healthier fats.

The American Diabetes Association guidelines recommend that you eat less than 10% of your calories from saturated fat, eat as little trans fat as possible, and consume no more than 300 milligrams of cholesterol per day. Get the remainder of your fat calories from the healthier monounsaturated and polyunsaturated fats. According to the American Diabetes Association nutrition recommendations, research does not support using omega-3 supplements (fish oil) for the prevention or treatment of heart attacks or strokes. Try to consume omega-3 fatty acid (EPA and DHA) and omega-3 linolenic acid (ALA) from fish, particularly fatty fish, at least two times (two servings) each week.

Fat affects blood glucose by slowing down the rise of blood glucose after you eat. In other words, a high-fat meal may cause a slower rise in blood glucose than a high-carbohydrate meal. This should not encourage you to eat a lot of fat, especially saturated fat, as a way to manage your blood glucose. Saturated fat has been shown to increase insulin resistance, which is common in prediabetes and type 2 diabetes. Maintain a moderate total fat intake, and eat the healthiest fats you can.

CHAPTER 4

Sodium, Potassium, and Blood Pressure Control

What's Ahead?

➡ Connection between high blood pressure and diabetes.
➡ Recommendations for blood pressure and sodium intake.
➡ Differences between salt and sodium and how to decrease both.
➡ The role of potassium in blood pressure control and how to eat more of it.
➡ More lifestyle changes to lower high blood pressure.

Diabetes and High Blood Pressure

According to the Centers for Disease Control (CDC), nearly three-quarters of adults (18 years old or older) with diabetes have high blood pressure, defined as greater than or equal to 140/90 mmHg, or are taking medication to lower blood pressure. Many people with prediabetes also have high blood pressure. In addition,

African Americans and people who are overweight are more likely to have high blood pressure. Years of uncontrolled high blood pressure can damage large blood vessels and result in heart disease or strokes, which account for nearly two-thirds of the deaths in people with diabetes. High blood pressure for years can also damage the body's small blood vessels and be a contributor to diabetes-related eye, nerve, and kidney disease.

The B in the diabetes ABC goals stands for blood pressure. The American Diabetes Association recommends that your blood pressure stay at or below 140/90 mmHg. Blood pressure control is just as critical to preventing diabetes complications as control of blood glucose (A for A1C) and cholesterol (C for Cholesterol)—or really all blood lipids.

Making some changes in your food choices, losing a few pounds (if needed), and making other lifestyle changes can help you control your blood pressure. In addition, many people with diabetes need to take one or more medications to control and maintain their blood pressure.

Sodium

Consuming less sodium has been shown to lower blood pressure in people with and those without diabetes who have high blood pressure. It's estimated that Americans eat about 3,400 milligrams of sodium a day; about three-quarters of this sodium is from processed foods. A handful of foods with a moderate amount of sodium, referred to as The Salty Six by the American Heart Association, contribute a large percent of the sodium we eat: breads and rolls, cold cuts and cured meats, pizza, poultry, soups, and sandwiches. That's simply because of the amounts of these foods we eat, some of which we purchase at supermarkets and others at restaurants. Restaurant foods, depending on the types of restaurants you go to and the foods you order, can contribute quite a bit of sodium to your eating plan. Learn about healthy restaurant eating in chapter 22.

As for Salt

Sodium and salt are different. Salt is composed of sodium chloride, which contains about 40% sodium and 60% chloride. One-quarter of a teaspoon of salt contains 575 milligrams (mg) of sodium. The salt you add during cooking and at the table (at home or in restaurants) contributes about 10% of the sodium we eat.

How Much Sodium?

According to the American Diabetes Association nutrition recommendations, your sodium intake should be less than 2,300 milligrams per day. The Dietary Guidelines suggest that people who want to lower their blood pressure can benefit from taking in less than 1,500 milligrams of sodium per day. For people with both diabetes and high blood pressure, the American Diabetes Association now suggests that their sodium recommendation be individualized. It's worth noting that it's very difficult to achieve the recommended sodium intake.

Tips to Reduce the Sodium in Processed and Restaurant Foods

• Review the sodium content on the Nutrition Facts labels. Foods that have less than 140 mg per serving are low in sodium.

• Use more unprocessed, fresh foods. Buy fresh fruits and vegetables.

• Limit your use of ready-to-eat and processed foods, such as canned soup, cold cuts, cereals, hot dogs, frozen entrées, salad dressings, and packaged mixes.

• Choose fish, chicken, and meats that are not processed, smoked, or prepared with sauces or seasonings.

• Choose snack foods and crackers that contain less than 150–200 mg of sodium per serving.

- Choose frozen meals or fast foods that contain less than 600–800 mg of sodium per serving.

- Choose natural cheeses such as mozzarella or cheddar rather than processed cheeses.

- Limit condiments, such as soy and teriyaki sauce, olives, pickles, and low-fat salad dressing.

- Make your own salad dressings with a healthy oil, such as corn, safflower, canola, or soybean oil, or a blend of canola and soybean oil that's low in saturated fat. Add vinegar, mustard, fruit or vegetable juice, fresh ground pepper, garlic, and herbs.

- Limit how often you eat restaurant foods. When you do eat restaurant meals, avoid the special sauces on sandwiches and the pickles, use oil and vinegar rather than prepared salad dressing, and have fresh salads or cooked vegetables.

Tips to Use Less Salt

- Don't use salt in cooking. Get creative with herbs, spices, and seasonings to add flavor. Most of them are very low in sodium.

- Don't add salt to rice, pasta, or hot cereals, as the packaging suggests, when you cook them.

- Take the salt off the table.

It's worth noting that there's a major push coming from the U.S. government to make food manufacturers and restaurants lower the sodium content of their foods.

Research shows that slowly reducing the sodium in the diet over time gives people the opportunity to adjust their palates and make lasting changes.

About Potassium

Beyond eating less sodium, another step you can take to lower high blood pressure is to eat sufficient amounts of fruits, vegetables, whole grains, and low-fat dairy foods. Evidence for this comes from a large study called the DASH (Dietary Approaches to Stop Hypertension). It reported the effects of three different eating plans on blood pressure. The lowest-sodium group ate 1,500 mg a day, the intermediate group ate 2,400 mg a day, and the high-sodium group ate 3,600 mg a day. In the lowest-sodium group, people also ate ample amounts of potassium from healthy amounts of grains; low-fat, high-calcium dairy foods (3 servings per day); fruits (4–6 servings per day); and vegetables (3–6 servings per day). This group lowered their blood pressure the most.

Amazingly, the effect of the healthy eating plan was evident within one week and had the greatest effect on lowering blood pressure in just 2 weeks! You guessed it. We don't currently eat enough potassium. See Table 5.4 on page 53 for high-potassium foods.

It appears that sufficient potassium, at least 4,700 milligrams per day, can reduce the impact of too much sodium on blood pressure. It may also reduce the risk of developing kidney stones and decrease bone loss associated with aging. Potassium plays a role in the proper function of the heart and helps maintain good blood pressure. Many people with diabetes take potassium-sparing drugs like ACE inhibitors, so check with your health-care provider before significantly increasing your potassium intake.

Other Lifestyle Changes Help, Too

Make these lifestyle changes in addition to lowering sodium intake and increasing potassium intake:

• Eat more low-fat or fat-free dairy foods. They can help lower blood pressure because of their potassium and calcium content. Eat or drink the number of servings of low-fat or fat-free dairy foods you need each day. Read more in chapter 11.

- Be moderate with alcohol. A moderate amount of alcohol (one drink a day for women and two drinks a day for men) offers heart health benefits, but more is not necessarily better. Read more in chapter 16.

- Be physically active nearly every day. Regular exercise can help prevent or control high blood pressure, and it can help you reduce your risk of heart disease. Another plus: exercise can help support weight loss and help you keep the pounds off. When people lose weight, they can often be more physically active, which burns more calories. Yes! A positive cycle!

- Lose a few pounds. Research shows that losing just 10 pounds can lower blood pressure regardless of other changes. Weight loss has the greatest effect on blood pressure in people who are overweight and already have high blood pressure.

- Don't smoke. If you do smoke, quit. Smoking cigarettes has been shown to injure blood vessel walls and speed up the process of hardening of the arteries. Even though smoking doesn't directly cause high blood pressure, it's not healthy for anyone, especially if you have high blood pressure and diabetes.

- Diagnose and treat sleep apnea. Sleep apnea is a chronic condition and is defined as having one or more pauses in breathing or shallow breaths while sleeping. The pauses can last from a few seconds to minutes and may occur numerous times each hour. Typically, normal breathing then starts again, sometimes with a loud snort or choking sound. Sleep apnea, which a significant number of people with prediabetes and type 2 diabetes have, can lead to high blood pressure as well as type 2 diabetes. Sleep apnea often goes undetected and untreated. If you have signs and symptoms of sleep apnea, such as snoring, being tired during the day, and irregular breathing during sleep, talk with your health-care provider about getting a sleep study done. If you have sleep apnea, treat it.

High blood pressure and diabetes are frequent companions. Take slow and steady steps to get and keep your blood pressure under control, from thinking about what and how much you eat to other lifestyle changes. Nearly all of these changes can help you improve your ABCs.

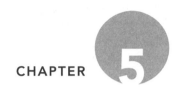

CHAPTER 5

Vitamins, Minerals, and Dietary Supplements

What's Ahead?

➡ Vitamins, minerals, and dietary supplements defined.
➡ American Diabetes Association recommendations on vitamins, minerals, and dietary supplements.
➡ How to get your vitamins and minerals from nutrient-dense foods and why.
➡ Top 10 food sources for five key vitamins and minerals.
➡ Facts about dietary supplements and what to consider before you try them.

Vitamins, Minerals, and Dietary Supplements Defined

Vitamins and minerals are essential nutrients for good health. These nutrients provide no calories. They're contained within foods and are essential for myriad functions and actions the body performs. To an extent, vitamins and minerals help the body use the food you eat to make it function. Each vitamin and mineral performs a unique task. In fact, beyond the vitamins and minerals that have been identified over the years as being essential for health, there are also hundreds of other substances in foods that remain unidentified by name or function. This is one reason why studies repeatedly show it's best to get your vitamins and minerals by eating a wide variety of foods.

Dietary supplements include vitamins, minerals, herbs, botanicals, and other substances that perform—or claim to perform—actions in your body to achieve good health or prevent or control health problems. The intention of supplements is just that: use them *in addition to* food, not as a *replacement* for healthy food choices.

In the U.S., the Food and Drug Administration (FDA) regulates dietary supplements, but it doesn't regulate the approval or marketing of supplements in the same manner as prescribed medicines. By law the FDA does not approve dietary supplements before they're allowed on the market, but it can take dietary supplements off the market if problems are reported. The FDA now requires all supplement containers to be labeled as a "dietary supplement" and to have a Supplement Facts label that is similar in look, but not content, to the Nutrition Facts label on foods and beverages.

Setting Vitamin and Mineral Recommendations for All

Vitamin and mineral deficiencies, which can result in diseases, were much more common several hundred years ago. Today, people in developed nations don't often get scurvy from having insufficient vitamin C, beriberi from a deficiency of thiamine, or rickets from not getting enough vitamin D. For the past few decades, U.S. government agencies and government-appointed experts have worked to establish which vitamins and minerals are necessary for health and the amounts of these vitamins and minerals people need at various ages and stages of life. These recommendations are based on the Dietary Reference Intakes (DRIs), developed with experts under the Institute of Medicine (IOM) at the National Academy of Sciences (NAS). Over time, the DRIs are reviewed and revised based on the evolving nutrition science.

What Does the American Diabetes Association Say?

If you eat a wide variety of nutrient-packed healthy foods, eat at least 1,200 calories a day, and generally keep your blood glucose within target goals, the American Diabetes Association does not recommend vitamins, minerals, or dietary supplements to achieve optimal nutrition and health.

A person with diabetes who meets any of the criteria below may need a specific vitamin or mineral supplement:

- Strict vegetarian/vegan (meaning you eliminate foods from several groups, including animal-based proteins and dairy foods, from your diet).

- Those following a weight-reducing meal plan of less than 1,200 calories per day.

- Pregnant or breast-feeding women.

- Elderly individuals.

If any of these factors apply to you, talk to your health-care provider about which if any vitamins and minerals you may need.

Missing Vitamins and Minerals

Many American adults and children don't get adequate amounts of several key nutrients mainly because they don't eat sufficient amounts of nutrient-dense foods. Nutrition intake surveys conducted by the U.S. government on a regular basis point out that while people generally eat more calories per day than ever (about 2,500 for men and 1,800 for women), we're falling short on certain key vitamins and minerals. The reason? We don't eat enough whole grains, fruits, and vegetables and eat too much added sugars and fat from refined grains, sugar-sweetened beverages, and sweets.

According to the Dietary Guidelines, the majority of Americans, regardless of age or sex, don't consume enough of these nutrients: vitamin A, vitamin D, vitamin E, folate (folic acid), vitamin C, calcium, potassium, and dietary fiber. Adolescent girls and women of child-bearing age are generally falling short on iron and folic acid. Additionally, adults over the age of 50 often don't get enough vitamin B_{12}.

Speaking of B_{12}, there's been some concern about vitamin B_{12} deficiency among people with prediabetes and type 2 diabetes who take the very commonly used blood glucose–lowering medication metformin. Evidence from the Diabetes Prevention Program Outcome Study (discussed on page 10–11) found a small increase in vitamin B_{12} deficiency among people who had taken metformin long term. This finding was not viewed as a significant concern.

Take a Foods-First Approach

Plan your meals and snacks so that you eat a wide variety of nutrient-dense foods, and get the majority of your vitamins and minerals from the foods you eat. If your calorie level is low (1,200 calories and below), you'll need to work even harder to carefully choose your foods and plan your meals to eat all the nutrients you need. After this move, if you still have some "nutrition gaps," consider taking a multivitamin and mineral supplement that offers an array of vitamins and minerals. However, it's difficult to get sufficient amounts of some vitamins and minerals from foods and multivitamin supplements. For these nutrients, such as calcium and vitamin D, you may need to take an individual supplement. (Read about Daily Values below.)

Get Your Fill of Vitamins and Minerals

While the vitamin and mineral needs of people with diabetes are no different from those of other people, research shows that many adults don't get enough of the essential vitamins and minerals.

Try these tips:

- Eat more fruits and vegetables, and eat a wide variety of them. Go for the high-color ones because they often provide more vitamins and minerals: orange, dark green, blue, and red.

- Eat more fruits and vegetables raw, unprocessed, or minimally processed.

- Make many of your starch choices whole wheat or whole grains: cereals and breads, brown rice, whole-wheat pasta, bulgur, and barley.

- Use legumes (beans, peas, and lentils) frequently. Make soups or bean salads, or sprinkle beans or peas on tossed salad. These foods are packed with vitamins and minerals.

- Eat or drink 2–3 servings a day of fat-free or low-fat milk, yogurt, or cheese. Most people don't get enough calcium and vitamin D. Dairy foods naturally contain calcium and are nearly always forti-fied with vitamin D.

See the individual chapters in section 2 for more tips on how to eat your vitamins and minerals.

Daily Values on the Nutrition Facts Label

The Nutrition Facts label uses the term "Daily Value (DV)" to pro-vide nutrient levels based on a calorie intake of 2,000 calories a day. This may be more or fewer calories than you need each day. The DVs, or percent DV (%DV), of a food are based on the govern-ment's recommendations for key nutrients. The DVs provide food manufacturers with guidelines to follow for food labeling and nu-trition claims. Table 5.1 lists current Daily Values and the amount

TABLE 5.1	Daily Values for Vitamins and Minerals with Levels for "Excellent Source" and "Good Source" Claims		
Nutrient	Daily Value (based on 2,000 calories/day)	Excellent Source (20% or higher)	Good Source (10–19%)
Dietary fiber	25 g	5 g	2.5–4.75 g
Sodium	2,400 mg	480 mg	240–456 mg
Potassium	3,500 mg	700 mg	350–665 mg
Vitamin A	5,000 IU	1,000 IU	500–950 IU
Vitamin C	60 mg	12 mg	6–11 mg
Calcium	1,000 mg	200 mg	100–190 mg
Iron	18 mg	3.6 mg	1.8–3.4 mg
Vitamin D	400 IU	80 IU	40–76 IU
Vitamin E	30 IU	6 IU	3–5.7 IU
Vitamin K	80 mcg	16 mcg	8–15.2 mcg
Thiamin	1.5 mg	0.3 mg	0.15–0.29 mg
Riboflavin	1.7 mg	0.34 mg	0.17–0.32 mg
Niacin	20 mg	4 mg	2–3.8 mg
Vitamin B_6	2 mg	0.4 mg	0.2–0.38 mg
Folate	400 mcg	80 mcg	40–76 mcg
Vitamin B_{12}	6 mcg	1.2 mcg	0.6–1.14 mcg
Biotin	300 mcg	60 mcg	30–57 mcg
Pantothenic acid	10 mg	2 mg	1–1.9 mg
Phosphorus	1,000 mg	200 mg	100–190 mg
Iodine	150 mcg	30 mcg	15–29 mcg
Magnesium	400 mg	80 mg	40–76 mg
Zinc	15 mg	3 mg	1.5–2.9 mg
Copper	2 mg	0.4 mg	0.2–0.38 mg
Selenium	70 mcg	14 mcg	7–13.3 mcg
Manganese	2 mg	0.4 mg	0.2–0.38 mg
Chromium	120 mcg	24 mcg	12–22.8 mcg
Molybdenum	75 mcg	15 mcg	7.5–14 mcg
Chloride	3,400 mg	680 mg	340–646 mg

Note: g, grams; mg, milligrams; IU, International Units; mcg, micrograms.

of the vitamin or mineral that a food must have per serving to use the nutrition claim "excellent source of" or "good source of."

- The terms "excellent source of," "rich in," and "high" mean that a serving (noted on the food label) of the food provides 20% or more of the Daily Value of a vitamin or mineral.

- The terms "good source of," "contains," and "provides" mean that a serving of the food must provide 10–19% of the Daily Value of a vitamin or mineral.

Top 10 for Four Key Vitamins and Minerals

Tables 5.2 to 5.5 provide the top 10 food sources (based on one serving of food) for the nutrients that Americans are most lacking: vitamin D, calcium, potassium (read about potassium in chapter 4), and vitamin B_{12}. Another nutrient Americans are severely lacking in is dietary fiber (Table 3.1). At the top of each of the tables in this chapter, find the DV for each nutrient and the amount needed for a food to be considered an "excellent source" or "good source" of the nutrient. Use these tables to see how the foods you eat stack up. Try these foods to introduce new nutrient-dense foods into your eating plan. (Nutrient data for these charts was obtained from the U. S. Department of Agriculture (USDA) nutrient database, a searchable database of over 8,000 foods at ndb.nal.usda.gov.)

TABLE 5.2	Vitamin D: Top 10 Food Sources			
Food	Serving	Food Group	Amount (IU)	%DV
Swordfish, cooked	3 oz	Protein	566	142
Salmon, sockeye, cooked	3 oz	Protein	447	112
Sardines, canned in oil	3 oz	Protein	164	41
Tuna, canned in water	3 oz	Protein	154	39
Orange juice, fortified	4 oz	Fruit	50	13
Milk, fat-free, fortified	8 oz	Milk	115	30
Milk, 1%, fortified	8 oz	Milk	98	25
Egg, whole, large (vitamin D found in yolk)	1	Protein	41	10
Cereal, dry flakes, fortified with 10% vitamin D	3/4 cup	Starch	30	8
Margarine, fortified	1 tsp	Fat	20	5

Daily Value = 400 IU
Excellent Source = 80 IU
Good Source = 40–76 IU

TABLE 5.3	Calcium: Top 10 Food Sources			
Food	Serving	Food Group	Amount (mg)	%DV
Milk, fat-free, calcium-fortified	1 cup	Milk	500	50
Milk, fat-free and 1% fat	1 cup	Milk	300	30
Soy beverage, calcium-fortified	1 cup	Milk	300	30
Buttermilk, fat-free	1 cup	Milk	285	29
Yogurt, low-fat plain	2/3 cup	Milk	325	33
Cheese, hard	1 oz	Protein	300–330	30–33
Ricotta cheese, skim	2 oz	Protein	170	17
Salmon, canned with bones	3 oz	Protein	180–210	18–21
Greens: collards, kale, spinach, turnip	1/2 cup	Vegetable	90–100	9–10
Custard or pudding	1/2 cup	Sweet	50	5

Daily Value = 1,000 mg
Excellent Source = 200 mg
Good Source = 100–190 mg

TABLE 5.4	**Potassium: Top 10 Food Sources**			
Food	Serving	Food Group	Amount (mg)	%DV
Beet greens, cooked	1/2 cup	Vegetable	655	19
White beans, cannellini	1/2 cup	Starch	595	17
Yogurt, fat-free plain	2/3 cup	Milk	416	12
Clams, canned	3 oz	Protein	534	15
Halibut, cooked	3 oz	Protein	490	14
Winter squash	1/2 cup	Starch	448	13
Spinach, cooked	1/2 cup	Vegetable	419	12
Tomato sauce	1/2 cup	Vegetable	405	12
Sweet potato, cooked	1/2 cup	Starch	3,475	14
Potato, cooked	1/2 cup	Starch	296	8

Daily Value = 3,500 mg
Excellent Source = 700 mg
Good Source = 350–665 mg

TABLE 5.5	**Vitamin B$_{12}$: Top 10 Food Sources**			
Food	Serving	Food Group	Amount (mcg)	%DV
Clams, cooked	3 oz	Protein	84	1400
Rainbow trout, wild, cooked	3 oz	Protein	5.4	90
Salmon, cooked	3 oz	Protein	4.8	80
Beef, top sirloin, cooked	3 oz	Protein	1.4	23
Breakfast cereals, fortified with vitamin B$_{12}$	1/2 cup	Starch	1.5–6	25–100
Milk, fat-free and 1% fat	1 cup			
Yogurt, plain, fat-free	2/3 cup	Milk	1	17
Cheese, Swiss	1 oz	Protein	0.95	16
Egg, cooked	1 large	Protein	0.6	10
Chicken breast, cooked	3 oz	Protein	0.3	5

Daily Value = 6.0 mcg
Excellent Source = 1.2 mcg
Good Source = 0.6–1.14 mcg

More on Dietary Supplements

Research shows that people with diabetes are more likely to take dietary supplements than the general public. Millions of dollars are spent purchasing dietary supplements each year, even though many have not been scientifically proven to provide health benefits. There is still too little research on the use and potential benefits of dietary supplements in general and in people with diabetes.

According to federal law, the Dietary Supplement Health and Education Act of 1994 (DSHEA), dietary supplements don't require FDA approval prior to being available on the market. Although there are effective dietary supplements on the market, this lack of prior approval leads to the marketing of many ineffective products and unfounded product claims. A number of dietary supplements are formulated specifically for and marketed directly to people with diabetes. If you choose to use dietary supplements, make sure your purpose for using them is sound and is factored in with the entirety of your diabetes care plan. Make sure your health-care providers know about the types and doses of dietary supplements you take and when you make a change. Purchase high-quality supplements. Learn more at the end of this chapter.

Table 5.6 is a list of some of the dietary supplements that have been researched or reviewed in animal and human studies for people with diabetes. More research is needed on most before any recommendation is warranted. Current American Diabetes Association nutrition recommendations don't recommend the use of dietary supplements for most people.

Before you buy dietary supplements, consider the following:

- Be aware that even the recommended dose of a supplement can cause side effects. Some supplements also interact with other supplements or prescribed medicines, so be sure to discuss the use of supplements with your health-care provider.

- If you have gaps in your nutrition, buy multivitamin and mineral supplements made by a reputable manufacturer, but continue to try to eat a wide variety of healthy foods to get your proper fill of nutrients.

TABLE 5.6 Dietary Supplement Information and Guidance

Vitamin, mineral, or dietary supplement name	Information and guidance
Antioxidants, like vitamins E, C, and A (as beta carotene and other carotenoids and selenium)	• Get recommended amounts of these nutrients through food sources. • Taking more of these nutrients is not beneficial. Research with large doses has even shown evidence of harm (vitamin E, carotene, and other antioxidants).
Alpha-lipoic acid (ALA)	• Some studies have shown that, in people with type 2 diabetes, ALA may help the muscles use glucose more efficiently and may make tissues more sensitive to the insulin made by the body. • Some studies have also found ALA to lessen the pain of diabetes nerve disease (neuropathy).
Chromium	• Chromium, in the form of chromium picolinate, may help lower blood glucose levels and improve blood lipids in people with type 2 diabetes who may be chromium deficient; however, the research is conflicting and doesn't confirm the need.
Cinnamon (the spice)	• Several small studies have shown that significant amounts of cinnamon consumed per day can lower blood glucose and A1C levels; however, a large review shows insufficient evidence to support its use.
Fenugreek	• Fenugreek is a legume (bean) that is high in fiber. In sufficient amounts, a few studies show it may lower blood glucose levels by slowing the rate at which foods with carbohydrates are broken down. In general, studies have not proven its effectiveness.
Garlic	• As a dietary supplement, garlic has been studied as an antioxidant and for its effect on lowering blood glucose by increasing the release of insulin, lowering blood pressure, and improving blood lipids. The research remains inconclusive.
American ginseng	• American ginseng is one of several species of ginseng plants and is the subject of most of the positive diabetes-related research. Lower blood glucose is the main benefit, but research is inconclusive.

continued

TABLE 5.6	*continued*
Vitamin, mineral, or dietary supplement name	**Information and guidance**
Magnesium	• The research on providing magnesium as a dietary supplement to improve blood glucose is mixed and inconclusive. • American adults and children generally don't get enough magnesium due to insufficient intake of high-magnesium foods, such as nuts, beans, yogurt, and spinach.
Vitamin D	• Consume the amount of vitamin D recommended in the Dietary Reference Intakes (Table 5.1). Research on the use of vitamin D supplementation for diabetes remains inconclusive and conflicting.
Coenzyme Q10 (ubiquinone)	• Coenzyme Q10, often referred to as CoQ10, is a frequently used supplement in people with diabetes because it's believed to improve various cardiovascular risk factors.
Turmeric	• Turmeric is a spice recognized for its anti-inflammatory properties. Research has shown that it may help prevent type 2 diabetes. Due to its anti-inflammatory actions, the supplement should be stopped at least 2 weeks before surgery to prevent excessive bleeding.
Vinegar	• A few studies have shown that 2 teaspoons of vinegar (any type) taken as part of a meal may decrease blood glucose levels following the meal. To date, there has not been enough research on vinegar to provide any kind of recommendation.

• Buy high-quality products. Look for USP, NF, TruLabel, or Consumer Labs on the label. These names indicate that you're buying a product that has been independently tested by a reputable lab. Buy products that have an expiration date.

- Continue to take your blood glucose–lowering medicines and other medications in your prescribed doses. If you think a dietary supplement may be lowering your blood glucose levels too much, tell your health-care providers and ask what changes they suggest. Do keep in mind that your prescription blood glucose–lowering medicines, taken in the correct doses, are more likely to reliably and more effectively lower your blood glucose compared with less well-researched dietary supplements.

- Spend your money wisely. If you want to try a supplement, choose one that has been extensively researched and demonstrates the greatest incidence of positive results.

- Use the Supplement Facts label, required on all dietary supplements, to learn more about the product before you buy it.

- Start one supplement at a time. Take it in the recommended dose, and take it for a month to see if it does what it promises.

Always tell your health-care providers about the dietary supplements you take, or ask them about supplements you want to take before you purchase or start taking them. They might advise you not to take a particular supplement, or they might ask you to stop taking one before surgery or another medical procedure. If they don't know you take them, they can't offer advice to keep you safe.

Learn More

American Diabetes Association: Guide to Herbs and Nutritional Supplements, by Laura Shane-McWorter, PharmD, BCPS, FASCP, BC-ADM, CDE, published by the American Diabetes Association.

Office of Dietary Supplements at National Institutes of Health: http://ods.od.nih.gov.

Food and Drug Administration: www.fda.gov/food/ dietarysupplements/default.htm.

6

Personalize Your Healthy Eating Plan

What's Ahead?

→ Create a healthy eating plan based on your lifestyle.
→ Find the best calorie range for you.
→ Know how many servings from each food group to eat each day.
→ Learn how to divide your food servings into meals and snacks.
→ Review sample meal plans for five calorie ranges.

The Right Calories for You

Do you wonder how many calories you need each day? The answer depends on many factors, including:

• Your age and sex.

• How active you are.

- Whether you want to lose or gain weight or stay the same weight.

- Whether you have lost and gained weight many times or this is your first effort.

- And more . . .

Table 6.1 can help you figure out how many calories and servings of various types of foods you need to eat each day. Servings of food, for the purposes of this book, are defined in the tables provided at the end of most of the chapters in section 2. These are based on the nutrient data used to develop the educational booklet **Choose Your Foods: Food Lists for Diabetes,** which was developed by diabetes nutrition experts and published by the American Diabetes Association and the Academy of Nutrition and Dietetics. Note that these food servings may be the same as or different from those used on the Nutrition Facts labels of food packages or other serving definitions.

These eating plans contain about 45–50% of calories from carbohydrate, 18–22% from protein, and 30–35% of calories from fat. These percentages fall into the ranges recommended by the Dietary Reference Intakes for the general public listed in Table 3.3 and reflect how many people divide up their calories. This is a mix of carbohydrate, protein, and fat that can help you meet your nutrition goals if you regularly choose nutrient-dense foods.

Here are some other factors to consider when you zero in on a range of calories that is best for you:

- **Activity level.** A sedentary lifestyle is defined as one in which the only physical activity you get is that needed to complete the daily tasks of life, such as getting to work, doing laundry, and fixing meals. An active lifestyle includes the activities of daily living plus regular physical activity (equal to walking more than 3 miles a day at 3–4 miles per hour).

- **Small stature, sedentary lifestyle.** If you are a small-stature, older woman who is sedentary, you may need no more than 1,200 calories a day to lose weight. At this calorie level, you may need a vitamin and mineral supplement to meet your nutrition needs. Discuss this with your health-care provider.

- **The servings and calculations for the milks and yogurts group are based on fat-free milk.** Children between 9 and 18 years of age need 1,300 mg of calcium per day. They should get at least 3 servings of milk per day. Adults aged 19–50 need 1,000 mg of calcium per day, which can be met with 2 servings of milk a day plus another serving of a high-calcium food. Women over age 50 need 1,200 mg of calcium per day. If you don't include milk or milk substitutes in your eating plan, discuss how to get the missing nutrients you need with a dietitian or health care provider. To make up for the carbohydrate in 1 cup of milk, add about 12–15 grams of carbohydrate from starches, non-starchy vegetables, or fruit.

- **Calorie and nutrient information for the foods in the protein group are based on an average of the amount of protein and fat in 1 ounce of lean protein foods (7 grams of protein and 2 grams of fat) or 1 ounce of medium-fat protein foods (7 grams of protein and 5 grams of fat), depending on which type of protein source you eat.** Adjust the grams or servings of fat based on the type of meats you tend to eat. Choose lean sources of protein foods as often as possible (see chapter 12 for more information) to eat less total fat, saturated and trans fat, and cholesterol.

Be Realistic! Aim for a Calorie Range

Your actual day-to-day calorie count doesn't need to add up to the same exact number every day; it greatly depends on the amounts of fat in the foods you eat. One day, your calorie count might be on the low side because you chose grilled chicken or fish and ate vegetables with little to no added fats. The next day, because you ate dinner out and chose a petite sirloin and shared a piece of apple pie, your calorie count is higher.

Another BIG factor in your daily calorie count is the accuracy of your portions. Research shows that people guesstimate portions too often and aren't accurate or necessarily honest with themselves. Calorie counts can be off by up to 500 calories at the end of each day simply due to eating a little more than you realized or guessing portions rather than weighing and measuring them. (Consider trying to precisely measure and weigh portions at least once a week, especially as you get started, then do so on occasion. Doing this will help "calibrate" your visual portion calculations.) Your main goal, over the course of a week or month, is to have your average intake match your target calories.

The Food Groups

This book groups foods into the six main groups used in the booklet **Choose Your Foods: Food Lists for Diabetes.** Foods are divided into these groups based on the nutrients they provide. Grouping foods this way makes it easier for you to plan, assemble, and eat healthy meals. Chapters in section 2 provide much more detail.

- **Starches:** This group includes grains such as bread, hot and dry cereal, rice, pasta, and crackers and starchy vegetables like potatoes, corn, peas, and legumes (beans). Eat at least three servings of whole grains or foods made with whole grain 3 day. Also, try to pack plenty of dietary fiber into the starches you choose.

- **Fruits:** This group includes all fresh, frozen, canned, and dried fruits and fruit juices made with 100% juice.

- **Milks and yogurts:** This group includes milk of all types, including cow's, soy, and rice milk, plus most yogurts. These foods are your best sources of calcium. Other dairy products that contain little or no calcium and mainly fat, such as cream cheese, cream, and butter, are generally found in the fat group. Find cheese, another source of calcium, in the protein group.

TABLE 6.1 **Find Your Calorie Range and Servings from Food Groups**

Which category fits you?	Women who . . . • want to lose weight • are small in stature • are sedentary	Women who . . . • are older and smaller stature • are larger stature and want to lose weight • are sedentary	Women who . . . • are moderate to large stature Men who . . . • are older • are small to moderate stature and want to lose weight	Children, teen girls, and women who . . . • are larger stature and active Men who . . . • are small to moderate stature and are at desired body weight	Teen boys and men who . . . • are active and moderate to large stature
Daily calorie ranges	1,200–1,400	1,400–1,600	1,600–1,900	1,900–2,300	2,300–2,800
Calculate Your Number of Servings from Each Food Group					
Starches	5	6	7	10	13
Vegetables (nonstarchy)	4	4	4	5	5
Fruits	2	2	3	3	4
Milks and yogurts	2	2	2	2	2
Protein	5 oz	6 oz	7 oz	8 oz	9 oz
Fats and oils	5	6	7	8	12
Percentage of calories and grams from carbohydrate, protein, and fat in eating plans					
Carbohydrate (grams)	150	165	195	244	304
Carbohydrdate (% of calories)	46	44	45	47	47
Protein (grams)	74	84	94	102	118
Protein (% of calories)	22	22	22	20	18
Fat (grams)	46	57	65	78	60
Fat (% of calories)	32	34	33	33	35

- **Vegetables (nonstarchy):** This group includes all fresh, frozen, and canned vegetables and vegetable juices. Starchy vegetables are in the starch food group.

- **Protein:** This group includes meats, poultry, seafood, eggs, cheese, peanut butter, and more. These foods provide you with the most concentrated sources of protein in your eating plan. Protein foods contain a wide range of fat, from nearly none in some white fishes to a good bit of fat in full-fat cheeses. Nuts and seeds are in the fat group because they contain more calories from fat than protein.

- **Fats and oils:** This group includes all sources and types of fats and oils, from the less healthy to the healthier. Foods like nuts, seeds, olives, and avocado are in this list.

A few other food groups are also covered in section 2:

- Sweets, desserts, and other carbohydrates.

- Non alcoholic beverages.

- Alcoholic beverages.

- Combination, convenience, and free foods.

From Servings to Meals and Snacks

The next step is to figure out how to divide your allotted calories and servings of food into balanced and tasty meals and snacks (if you need and want snacks). Eating three square meals a day is the foundation of a healthy eating plan that can help you keep your blood glucose under control, especially if you take a blood glucose–lowering medicine that can cause low blood glucose.

Many people often skip breakfast. Yet breakfast is an important meal for a few reasons. First, it's an easy meal to fit in a serving or two of the foods we don't eat enough of—whole grains, fruit, nuts, and seeds, which tend to be harder to find if you eat out. Second, some research shows that people who've lost weight and kept it off regularly eat breakfast. Last, eating a healthy breakfast can have a purely psychological benefit; the positive action can kick your day off on a healthy note and power up your resolve to eat healthy the rest of the day.

To snack or not to snack? People with diabetes used to be told to eat every few hours to make sure their blood glucose didn't drop into the hypoglycemic range (below 70 mg/dL), so they ate snacks at regular intervals. These instructions were provided. Times have changed dramatically!

Reason one: today we have a host of newer blood glucose–lowering medications that don't generally cause hypoglycemia. These are often the initial medications, like metformin, that people with type 2 diabetes are prescribed. Reason two: diabetes meal planning is less focused on rules and more focused on encouraging you to find an eating and lifestyle plan that is flexible and works for you. Some people find they want or need snacks as part of their day-to-day eating plan to control between-meal hunger and be more successful with weight control. Other people don't want to be bothered with snacking during the day. They're happy to eat three meals a day.

Bottom line: snacks are no longer required. Read through this checklist to determine if you want to include snacks in your eating plan or not:

- Snacks help you eat the correct amounts of foods at your meals and decrease between-meal hunger.

- Snacks prevent low blood glucose levels between meals, even after you and your health-care provider have adjusted your blood glucose–lowering medications to prevent hypoglycemia.

- Snacks help you meet your calorie needs (especially for young children, women who are pregnant, or people who are underweight or recovering from a medical problem or procedure).

- Snacks help you eat enough of certain nutrients because of the types of foods you eat at snacks, such as yogurt, fruit, vegetables, or nuts.

Assemble Your Eating Plan

Ask yourself these questions about your daily life to help you identify the types of foods you want in your eating plan:

- What foods do you enjoy, and when do you want to eat them?

- When do you take your blood glucose–lowering medications, and is this working for you based on your current life schedule and lifestyle (if not, discuss with your health-care provider)?

- How often and at what times do you have low blood glucose (hypoglycemia), if ever?

- How much food do you like to eat at your meals and snacks? Answers can differ for different meals.

- Do you want or need snacks?

- What other nutrients do you need to consider? For example, do you have concerns about sodium and blood pressure, or saturated and trans fat and blood lipids?

- How often do you eat meals away from home? What types of foods do you eat when you eat out?

- Do you take vitamin and mineral supplements? Which ones and how much?

- What is your weight history?

- What is your usual activity level? When do you usually do physical activity?

- What is your usual daily schedule? If you work, what are your work hours? How do your weekdays vary from weekends? Are there other regular events in your schedule to consider?

Learn by Example: Three Sample One-Day Meal Plans

These one-day sample meals for three calorie ranges can help you translate the calories and food servings in Table 6.1 into an eating plan that you can put into action. These sample meals include a wide variety of foods; some are foods you may prepare at home, others are convenience foods and restaurant foods.

SAMPLE MEAL PLAN: 1,200–1,400 CALORIES

Daily Servings from Food Groups

5 starch   2 fruit   2 milk   4 vegetable   5 oz protein   5 fat

BREAKFAST

1 cup oatmeal (cooked) with	2 starch
2 tsp ground flaxseed and	free food
1 Tbsp raisins	1/2 fruit
1/2 cup fat-free milk	1/2 milk
1/2 cup fat-free plain yogurt with	1/2 milk
1/2 medium banana, sliced (4 oz)	1/2 fruit

LUNCH

1/2 whole-wheat pita pocket (6 ")	1 starch
2 oz salmon (canned) made with	2 oz protein
2 tsp mayonnaise	2 fat
1/2 cup sliced cucumbers	1/2 vegetable
1/3 cup alfalfa sprouts	1/2 vegetable
1/4 avocado, sliced	1 fat
1 oz baked tortilla chips	1 starch
1 nectarine (5 oz)	1 fruit

DINNER

Chef salad	3 vegetable
2 cups mixed greens	
2 Tbsp chopped mushrooms	
2 Tbsp chopped peppers	
1/3 cup roasted beets	
1/3 cup diced tomatoes	

3 oz roasted chicken	3 oz protein
2 tsp canola oil	2 fat
Vinegar	free food
Dinner roll, whole wheat	1 starch

EVENING SNACK

1 pkg sugar-free hot cocoa mix made with 1/2 cup fat-free milk	1 milk

---

SAMPLE MEAL PLAN: **1,400–1,600 CALORIES**

Daily Servings from Food Groups

6 starch   2 fruit   2 milk   4 vegetable   6 oz protein   6 fat

BREAKFAST

1 whole grain bagel thin (2 oz) with	2 starch
1 1/2 Tbsp light cream cheese	1 fat
3/4 cup blueberries with	1 fruit
1/3 cup fat-free plain yogurt	1/2 milk

LUNCH

Tuna salad made with:

3 oz tuna (1/2 cup), water-packed	3 oz protein
1 Tbsp light mayonnaise	1 fat
2 Tbsp diced celery	1 vegetable
1 Tbsp diced onions	
Tomato slices and lettuce leaves	1 free food
1 whole-wheat tortilla	2 starch
1 cup baby carrots	1 vegetable
1 cup fat-free milk	1 milk

DINNER

3 oz grilled salmon with lemon and herbs	3 oz protein free food
Stir-fried vegetables with	
1/4 cup onions, cooked	2 vegetable
1/2 cup snow peas, cooked	
1/2 cup red peppers, cooked	
2 tsp canola oil	2 fat
2/3 cup brown rice	2 starch

EVENING SNACK

Mix together:

1/2 cup crushed canned pineapple (packed in own juice)	1 fruit
1/3 cup fat-free plain yogurt	1/2 milk
1/8 cup chopped pecans	2 fat

SAMPLE MEAL PLAN: 1,900–2,300 CALORIES

Daily Servings from Food Groups

10 starch   3 fruit   2 milk   5 vegetable   8 oz protein   8 fat

BREAKFAST

1 fried egg with	1 oz protein
2 tsp light tub margarine	1 fat
2 slices whole-wheat toast with	2 starch
2 tsp low-sugar jelly	free food
1/2 large grapefruit	1 fruit
1 cup fat-free milk	1 milk

LUNCH

Fast-food hamburger, plain (quarter pound)	2 starch, 3 oz protein, 2 fat
with ketchup and mustard	free food
1 order small french fries	2 starch, 2 fat
with ketchup	free food
1 garden salad (large) with	2 vegetable
1 tsp oil (2 fat) plus vinegar (free)	1 fat

DINNER

2 cups turkey chili (homemade)	3 starch, 1 vegetable, 3 oz protein
1 oz grated low-fat cheese	1 oz protein, 1 fat
1/2 cup baby carrots	1 vegetable
1/2 cup sliced cucumbers	1 vegetable
2 Tbsp light ranch salad dressing for dip	1 fat
1 sliced kiwi large (3 1/2 oz)	1 fruit

EVENING SNACK

1/4 cup low-fat granola (no raisins)	1 starch
2/3 cup fat-free plain yogurt	1 milk
1 cup raspberries	1 fruit

CHAPTER **7**

Secrets of Losing Weight and Keeping Pounds Off

What's Ahead?

➡ Realistic weight loss and maintenance goals.
➡ When weight loss will and won't improve your ABCs.
➡ Weight loss medications, surgery, and beyond.
➡ Successful strategies for weight loss.
➡ Successful strategies to keep weight off for good.

For people with prediabetes and type 2 diabetes, a major recommendation of the American Diabetes Association is to get to or stay at a healthy weight. Today, roughly two-thirds of American adults are overweight or obese. One-third are overweight and one-third are obese. Obese is defined as more than 30% above a desirable body mass index (BMI).

And too many children and adolescents are overweight and are at risk of or have developed prediabetes or type 2 diabetes.

As discussed in chapter 1, being overweight is a significant risk factor for prediabetes and type 2 diabetes.

During the past few decades, numerous research studies, large and small, have taught us a lot about the positive impact a small amount of weight loss (losing about 7% of total body weight) has on health: lowered blood pressure, improved blood lipids, increased mobility and fewer joint problems, decreased depression and sleep apnea, and more.

Identify Realistic Weight Loss and Maintenance Goals

For most people who are overweight or obese, it's neither realistic nor necessary to aim for the weight they were as a teen or young adult. Losing weight, and keeping the majority of the weight off, is tough for everyone for several reasons. Due to a number of hormonal and metabolic changes that impact hunger and appetite control, people who lose weight seem to need fewer calories to maintain their lighter weight. It also seems that the presence of insulin resistance, a reality for most people with prediabetes and type 2 diabetes, can make weight loss and control even tougher.

Research shows that most people are more successful if they set their initial weight loss goal at knocking off that first 7% of weight. Achieve that weight loss goal, see how it feels, and ask yourself whether you need to lose more weight to achieve your health goals. Weight loss studies (as discussed in Chapter 1) repeatedly show that the maximum weight loss for most people occurs between 6 months and 1 year of weight loss efforts.

Once you have achieved 7% weight loss, you should ask yourself, "Do I feel better? Have some of my ABC numbers improved? Have other health problems been minimized?" Then reflect on what has made you successful. What actions have you put in place? You'll need to keep these up to keep your weight down. Take some time to see if you can and how you will maintain this all-important 7% weight loss over time. Keeping off those initial pounds lost is important for your long-term health and control of your ABCs. The last thing you want to do after you've worked hard to lose weight is to go back to your old habits and put those pounds right back on again. Successful weight loss and maintenance means making your behavior and eating habit changes permanent.

If you find that you want to lose more weight, consider restarting your weight loss efforts several months after you've lost your initial 7% of body weight, so you know you can comfortably practice the healthy habits required for weight control.

Weight Loss and Improvements in Blood Glucose Control

Not very long ago diabetes experts thought type 2 diabetes was a pretty static condition. They thought most people could control their blood glucose with the combination of a healthy eating plan, some weight loss, and sufficient physical activity. Prediabetes was barely on the radar screen! Due to several long-term studies in people with type 2 diabetes, this notion has gone by the wayside for most people. Research has shown that type 2 diabetes progresses, and most people need to partner weight loss, healthy eating, and physical activity with a sufficient amount of blood glucose–lowering medication to achieve their diabetes management goals.

A minority of people with prediabetes or type 2 diabetes can— if they lose a lot of weight soon after their diagnosis of diabetes and keep it off—reverse their prediabetes or type 2 diabetes or put it into what's called remission. (See the discussion below about weight loss surgery.) That doesn't mean they'll never have to worry about diabetes. In fact, they should regularly have their A1C checked. Also, as people age, blood glucose levels tend to rise. Put all these factors together and it's quite likely type 2 diabetes may return.

For people diagnosed with type 2 diabetes after they've had it for a number of years, or a number of years pass before they start to work on losing weight, it's not likely that a realistic amount of weight loss will control blood glucose levels without the assistance of some blood glucose–lowering medication.

You can easily track your success with weight loss and blood glucose control by working with your provider. Research shows that you can start seeing positive changes in your glucose levels from weight loss anywhere from 6 weeks to 3 months after you start to change your lifestyle habits. If weight loss doesn't lower your glucose levels, then it's likely you'll need to take one or more glucose-lowering medications.

About Weight Loss Medications, Surgery, and Beyond

Beyond calorie reduction and increased physical activity, there is a quickly escalating number of weight loss medications. Four of these medications approved by the Food and Drug Administration (FDA) are Belviq, Qysmia, Contrave, and Saxenda (which is a larger dose of glucose-lowering medication in the category of GLP-1 analogs). There will likely be more medications to come. None are miracle cures. They're aids that can work if they're used in concert with calorie reduction and increased physical activity. Investigate these medications by discussing their upsides and downsides with your health-care provider.

Weight loss surgery, either the less invasive but less effective lap band procedure or one of the more invasive surgeries, like Roux-en-Y gastric bypass or sleeve gastrectomy, is an option for some people. Weight loss surgery can, for some people with prediabetes or type 2 diabetes, result in significant weight loss and improvements in blood glucose control. The success of the various surgeries regarding weight loss and remission of diabetes varies from case to case. If you are significantly overweight and continue to have a difficult time being successful with weight loss, you may want to explore weight loss surgery with your health-care provider.

The future promises various new nonsurgical technologies to minimize calorie intake and maximize weight loss. All will undergo extensive research by the developers and the FDA before they're approved by the FDA for use. Keep your eyes and ears open for news on these new technologies. Read what you can, and have an open dialog with your providers about new therapies that may help you achieve your diabetes goals.

Successful Strategies for Weight Loss and Keeping Pounds Off

By looking at the combined results of several long-term research studies, among them DPPOS and Look AHEAD (see chapter 1), as well as ongoing results from the National Weight Control Registry, the secrets of successful weight loss are emerging. Though there are commonalities in strategies to lose weight and keep it off, there are also some differences. Both losing weight and maintaining weight loss definitely require discipline and persistence.

Successful Strategies for Weight Loss

- Tackle your weight when you are ready, willing, and able. Do it for yourself, not your spouse, friends, or providers. This goal has to be your goal.

- Set a realistic and achievable weight loss goal.

- Take one step at a time. Slowly change your food habits with an eating plan that considers your food preferences.

- Focus on portions and portion control.

- Choose foods with less added sugars and fewer calories from fat. Fat is a concentrated source of calories.

- Eat foods that provide sufficient dietary fiber. They include fruits, vegetables, and whole grains.

- Start out by changing the behaviors that you are most ready and able to change.

- Get and stay physically active. Find something you enjoy doing and can easily incorporate into your lifestyle. Start slow, and work up to at least 30 minutes most days.

- Eat breakfast every day. It can get you off to a healthy start.

- Consider the use of meal replacements (bars, meals, soups, or drinks) that are calorie- and portion-controlled foods if you think they may offer you assistance.

- Watch less than 10 hours of TV per week, and minimize sedentary activity.

- Keep records about various aspects of your plan. Record keeping makes you accountable.

- Consider finding a weight management support group or program delivered by a credentialed health-care provider or trained facilitator. You may want to take advantage of a work- or community-based program or consider an online option. For people who have prediabetes, check out programs in your community or online that are delivering the research-based National Diabetes Prevention Program at this link: https://nccd.cdc.gov/DDT_DPRP/Registry.aspx.

- Experience some early weight loss. Studies show that early weight loss predicts later success. As the saying goes, success breeds success.

Successful Strategies for Keeping Pounds Off for Good

- Appreciate that you've got to continue to practice the behaviors you learned while losing weight. There is no going back to your old habits and way of eating. The physiologic reality is that you will need fewer calories to maintain your lower weight than you did when you were at this weight previously.

- Maintain a calorie-appropriate lower fat intake.

- Eat breakfast.

- Keep your eating plan simplified, and minimize your food choices.

- Practice restraint around foods that are unhealthy and high in calories.

- Get a sufficient amount of regular activity. Participants in the National Weight Control Registry report getting about 60 minutes a day.

- Minimize screen time, like watching TV or using a computer or other technology.

- Maintain frequent and ongoing contact with a health-care provider, behavioral counselor, or other support system that helped you lose weight. Remember, keeping lost weight off is the tough part.

- Have a relapse prevention plan ready. Put it in place if you gain a few pounds. Don't let gaining a few pounds turn into returning to your heavier weight.

- Weigh yourself regularly, at least weekly if not more often.

2

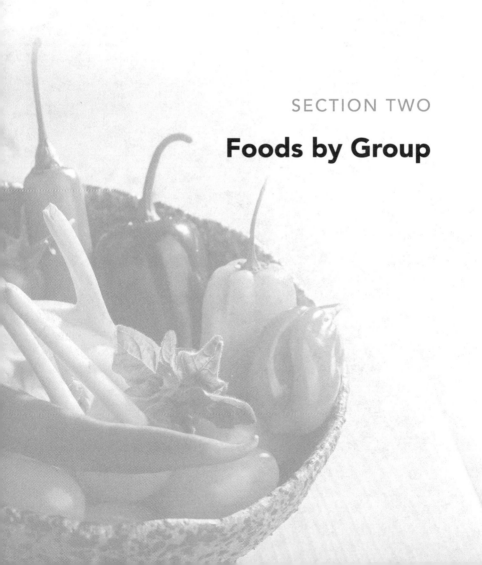

Foods by Group

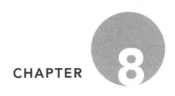

CHAPTER

Starches

What's Ahead?

- → The nutrition assets of starches.
- → Healthy eating goals for starches.
- → Assess the servings of starch you eat now.
- → The ideal number of starch servings for you.
- → Tips to help you buy, prepare, and eat more healthy starches.
- → Serving sizes and nutrition numbers for starches.

Foods in the Starch Group

Starches include all foods made from grains, such as breads, hot and dry cereals, rice, pasta, crackers, and grains like quinoa, millet, and barley. This group also contains starchy vegetables like potatoes, corn, green peas, and legumes (beans, peas, and lentils).

In general, starches provide you with a ready source of energy because they contain mainly carbohydrate. They're also good sources of some B vitamins, magnesium, copper, iron, selenium, and dietary fiber, if they're whole grain. The orange-colored starchy vegetables, such as sweet potatoes, winter squash, and pumpkin, are great sources of carotenoids (vitamin A). White potatoes are loaded with vitamin C. Also, white potatoes, sweet potatoes, and winter squash are full of potassium.

Green Light on Whole Grains

Studies show that eating more whole grains and dietary fiber can have both immediate and long-term health benefits. In the short term, eating more whole grains and fiber can minimize constipation and help you manage your weight by helping you feel fuller longer. In the long term, eating plans that contain whole grains decrease the risk for heart disease, prediabetes, type 2 diabetes, and colon cancer.

Whole grains contain the entire grain kernel: the bran, germ, and endosperm. Examples of whole grains are whole-wheat flour, whole-wheat pasta, oatmeal, corn (as cornmeal), quinoa, brown rice, barley, and millet. One serving of whole grain equals 16 grams of whole-grain ingredients. You see manufacturers boasting about the grams of whole grain on the front of their packaging. That's in part because they're bragging but for another important reason as well. Whole grains aren't a nutrient and therefore aren't identified on the Nutrition Facts label.

Grains that are no longer "whole" go through a refining process. This removes most of the bran and some of the germ, thereby removing some dietary fiber, vitamins, minerals, and micronutrients. Keep in mind that most refined grains in foods today are enriched. This means that certain B vitamins (such as thiamine, riboflavin, niacin, and folic acid) and iron are added back after processing. In fact, federal law requires that refined grains be enriched with folic acid to help prevent spina bifida, also called neural tube birth defects. Fiber, however, is not added back to refined grains.

Whole Grains versus Fiber

What's the difference between whole grains and fiber? Foods made with or containing whole grains contain some fiber. But fiber is in more foods than just whole grains, and there's more nutrition benefit to whole grains than just dietary fiber. Fiber is also found in fruits; starchy vegetables, such as corn and green peas; legumes, such as beans, peas, and lentils; and in nonstarchy vegetables, such as broccoli, green beans, and carrots. Fiber is covered in depth in chapter 3.

Starches Get Mixed Up with Fat and Sugar

Whole grains, legumes, and starchy vegetables can be very healthy, or they can be high in calories because they get loaded with added fat and sugars. Sometimes you add the fat when you prepare the food or before you eat it. Consider corn on the cob glistening with butter, pasta covered with cheese or cream sauce, or a bagel slathered with cream cheese. Sometimes manufacturers or restaurants add fat or sugar to the food before you eat it. Consider sweetened dry cereals, packaged sweetened oatmeal, fried snack foods, and glazed doughnuts. Very often, this added fat consists of too much unhealthy saturated and trans fats. It's a healthy eating challenge to figure out how to eat starches before they get mixed up with added fat and sugars.

Get to Know Yourself

If you want to change your eating habits, you need to take stock of your current eating habits. Ask yourself these questions about the starches you eat:

- How many starch servings do I eat on most days?

- What starches do I choose? Are any, a few, or all of them whole grains? Are they low, moderate, or high in fiber?

Healthy Potatoes?

Americans eat a lot of potatoes, and although potatoes are often maligned, potatoes on their own are quite nutritious and are a healthy choice for people with diabetes. But we love to load them with fat. Think about french fries, potato chips, or a baked potato loaded with sour cream and butter.

Consider how a healthy, naturally fat-free baked potato quickly becomes high in fat and calories:

1 medium (6 oz) baked potato = 160 calories, 0% calories from fat

+

2 tsp stick margarine = 90 calories, 100% calories from fat

+

2 Tbsp sour cream = 45 calories, 100% calories from fat

Now this baked potato has nearly 300 calories, and almost half of those calories come from fat.

- Do I eat enough whole grains (at least half of your starch servings)?

- Do the starches I choose have added fat and sugars in, on, or around them?

How Many Starch Servings for You?

In chapter 6, you determined which calorie range was best for you to follow at the moment. Find that calorie range in Table 6.1, and then spot the number of starch servings to eat each day. It should be somewhere between 5 and 13. You might be saying to yourself, "WOW, this seems like a lot," but think about your meals. For instance, you might make a sandwich with two slices of whole-grain bread. That's 2 starch servings for the bread and even more if you grab a handful of chips. Let's say that you have 2 cups of pasta. That's 6 starch servings and even more if you add some garlic bread. When you add up the starch servings, you may actually need to cut down a bit, or perhaps you've been cutting down too much.

Get to Know Your Serving Sizes

Table 8.1 at the end of this chapter (starting on page 92) shows serving sizes for many of the starch foods you commonly eat, along with their calories, carbohydrate, fat, and fiber. One starch serving contains an average of 15 grams of carbohydrate, 3 grams of protein, 1 gram of fat, and 80 calories.

In general, the serving size for 1 starch serving is:

- 1/2 cup of cooked cereal or starchy vegetable.
- 1/3 cup of cooked grain or pasta.
- 1 ounce of dry cereal.
- 1 ounce of bread (usually 1 slice).
- 3/4–1 ounce of most snack foods like pretzels and crackers.

To eat the number of calories you shoot for each day, it's important to eat the correct serving sizes. To hit your calorie and servings targets, weigh and measure your foods at least occasionally to make sure you're estimating correctly. Use the same bowls and cups to help you "eyeball" the proper amount. For example, always eat your cereal out of the same bowl or serve your pasta on the same size plate. If you currently serve your meals on big plates, you may consider using smaller plates so less food on your plate looks like more. It's a small change, but it can make a big difference!

Sample Meal Plans

The sample meal plan below gives you an idea of how to fit 6 starch servings into an eating plan with 1,400–1,600 calories a day. You'll see that the starch servings are in bold for quick identification.

Chapter 6 has sample plans and nutrition information for the other calorie ranges.

ONE-DAY MEAL PLAN: 1,400–1,600 CALORIES

BREAKFAST

1 whole-grain bagel thin (2 oz) with	**2 starch**
1 1/2 Tbsp light cream cheese	1 fat
3/4 cup blueberries with	1 fruit
1/3 cup fat-free plain yogurt	1/2 milk

LUNCH

Tuna salad made with	
3 oz tuna (1/2 cup), water-packed	3 oz protein
1 Tbsp light mayonnaise	1 fat
2 Tbsp diced celery	1 vegetable
1 Tbsp diced onions	
Tomato slices and lettuce leaves	1 free food
1 whole-wheat tortilla	2 starch
1 cup baby carrots	**1 vegetable**
1 cup fat-free milk	1 milk

DINNER

3 oz grilled salmon with	3 oz protein
lemon and herbs	free food
Stir-fried vegetables with	
1/4 cup onions, cooked	2 vegetable
1/2 cup snow peas, cooked	
1/2 cup red peppers, cooked	
2 tsp canola oil	2 fats
2/3 cup brown rice	**2 starch**

EVENING SNACK

Mix together:	
1/2 cup crushed canned pineapple (packed in own juice)	1 fruit
1/3 cup fat-free plain yogurt	1/2 milk
1/8 cup chopped pecans	2 fat

Healthy Starches Challenge

To choose healthier starches, you'll face a few challenges. Try to slowly change your eating habits and food choices by:

- Choosing starches with whole grains and fiber.
- Adding more healthy starches to your meals and snacks.
- Selecting starch toppings that are low in fat or fat-free.

Here are tips that can help you succeed.

Breads

- Choose breads that state at least 8 grams of whole grain on the package or state in the ingredients: 100% whole wheat, whole-grain [name of grain], whole wheat, stone-ground whole [name of grain]. Don't be fooled; wheat bread or bread that is brown in color isn't necessarily whole grain. It may be made with enriched wheat or simply contain molasses.

- Choose bread that contains at least 3 grams of fiber per slice. You might need to try a few different kinds to find one you enjoy.

- Choose a small whole-grain roll instead of a biscuit, scone, or croissant, which contain fat.

- Choose whole-grain tortillas, pizza crust, muffins, hot dog buns, and hamburger buns. They're all available in most grocery stores, with more brands likely on the way.

Crackers

- Choose low-fat or fat-free crackers made with whole grains rather than butter crackers made from enriched flour.

- Choose crackers with at least 2 grams of fiber per serving. More fiber is better.

continued

Cereals

- Pick whole-grain dry cereals made from bran that contain at least 3–5 grams of fiber per serving.

- Mix a few dry cereals together. Use one very high fiber cereal, like All-Bran, that contains 8 or more grams of fiber per serving, and then mix in small amounts of other whole-grain cereals you enjoy. Top your bowl of cereal with ground flax or chia seeds or a sprinkle of wheat germ. Each has their nutrition assets.

- Get a few extra grams of fiber from hot cereal by choosing oatmeal or oat bran rather than cream of wheat or grits. Cook it with ground flax or wheat germ. (Skip instant packaged cereals.)

- Consider new-to-you whole grains for hot cereal, like farro and quinoa. Make up a batch to serve for several breakfasts.

Grains, Including Rice and Pasta

- Choose brown rice, wild rice, or a mix of several types of rice instead of white rice.

- Opt for steamed brown rice instead of steamed or fried white rice in Chinese restaurants.

- Pick whole-wheat pasta. There are many on the market; you might need to try a few different kinds to find one you enjoy.

- Learn to prepare healthy whole grains: barley, bulgur, corn, farro, millet, oats, quinoa, wheat berries, whole-wheat couscous, and other less well-known grains. They're becoming more widely available in supermarkets, and you'll find tasty recipes for all of them.

- Use whole grains in soups, stews, salads, and stir-fries. Barley makes a great addition to vegetable soup, while quinoa and bulgur are popular additions to salads.

continued

Starchy Vegetables

- Keep frozen starchy vegetables like green peas, edamame, and corn in your freezer. Add them to soups, whole-grain pasta, or brown rice for a quick and easy meal.

- Mix pumpkin or squash purée into whole-grain waffle or pancake batter or macaroni and cheese casserole. (Consider 1/2 cup for a 4-person serving.) If you start with a mix for pancakes or waffles, make sure it contains whole grains, and use whole-grain macaroni or pizza.

Legumes (Beans, Peas, and Lentils)

- Drain and rinse canned beans to reduce the sodium content by up to 40%. Better yet, start with dry types.

- Enjoy vegetables and hummus, or other bean purées, as an afternoon snack.

Easy Ways to Eat More Healthy Starches

- In a meatloaf or meatball recipe, substitute whole-grain bread, bulgur, or brown rice for some of the meat.

- Add whole-wheat pasta, peas, or beans to a vegetable soup.

- Prepare a hearty bean or pea soup as a main course. Divide the leftovers into individual portions and store them in the freezer for a quick meal.

- Substitute whole-grain flour or cornmeal for half of the flour in pancake or waffle batter and in muffins or bread dough.

- When you cook a whole grain, make enough for extra servings through the week, or freeze a few servings. If you don't use the leftovers as a side dish, toss them on salads or into soups or casseroles. Mix in toasted nuts or dried fruit to make them even healthier.

- Eat whole-grain dry cereal without milk as a snack on the run, or mix it with yogurt and dried fruit for a healthy snack at home.

- Toss leftover cold corn, brown rice, bulgur, or green peas on a salad. (Entrée salads can become meals made in minutes and can contain myriad ingredients.)

- Open a can of garbanzo beans (chickpeas) or kidney beans and add them to a salad, tomato sauce, three-bean salad, or soup. Better yet, start with dry beans and cook them quickly in a pressure cooker. Freeze extras, and take them out as you need them.

- Choose lower-fat alternatives to the high-fat starches you currently eat (Table 8.2).

- Have whole-wheat pretzels or light popcorn for a snack.

- Use winter squash and sweet potatoes frequently. They are loaded with vitamin A.

TABLE 8.2	High-Fat Starches and Low-Fat Alternatives		
Food	**Serving**	**Calories**	**Fat (g)**
Muffin	3 oz	158	4
Bagel	*3 oz*	*178*	*2*
Croissant	1	109	6
Bread	*1 slice*	*65*	*1*
Potato chips	1 oz	152	10
Potato chips, baked	*1 oz*	*100*	*1*
French fries	Small order	230	10
Baked potato	*Small, 3 oz*	*98*	*0*
Taco shell	1	100	6
Tortilla, corn	*1*	*56*	*1*
Macaroni and cheese	6 oz	250	13
Spaghetti and tomato sauce	*6 oz*	*209*	*2*
Refried beans	1/2 cup	136	3
Refried beans, fat-free	*1/2 cup*	*93*	*0*

Low-fat alternatives are in italics.

Use Low-Fat or Fat-Free Starch Toppers

- Spread soft or light cream cheese on bagels or toast.

- Put reduced-calorie sour cream or plain yogurt mixed with fresh or dried herbs on baked potatoes.

- Put cottage cheese in the blender to make it smooth. Mix in herbs or seasonings to top pasta or baked potatoes.

- Put a tasty mustard on baked potatoes or sandwiches.

- Mix tomato sauce with whole-grain pasta or brown rice.

- Choose a tub margarine that has no trans fats.

- Use low-fat or fat-free mayonnaise on sandwiches.

- Put salsa on low-fat tortilla chips, Mexican burritos, or fajitas.

TABLE 8.1 Serving Sizes, Calories, and Nutrients for Starches

Food	Serving Size
BREADS	
Bagel, plain	1/4 large
Biscuit, baked	1 biscuit (2 1/2" dia)
Bread, French	1 slice
Bread, Italian	1 slice
Bread, pumpernickel	1 slice (5" x 4" x 3/8")
Bread, raisin	1 slice
Bread, reduced-calorie, light	2 slices
Bread, reduced-calorie, wheat	2 slices
Bread, reduced-calorie, white	2 slices
Bread, rye, light or dark	1 slice, thick
Bread, sourdough	1 slice
Bread, unfrosted cinnamon	1 slice
Bread, white	1 slice
Bread, whole-grain	1 slice
Bread, whole-wheat	1 slice
Chapati	1 oz
Ciabatta	1 oz
Cornbread, baked	1 1/2 oz
English muffin	1/2 muffin
Hamburger bun or roll	1/2 small bun
Hot dog bun or roll	1/2 bun
Naan	3 1/4" square
Pancake, plain, frozen, reheated	1 pancake (4" dia)
Pita bread, white	1/2 pita
Roll, plain, dinner	1 roll (1 oz)
Roti	1 oz
Sandwich flat buns, whole-wheat	1 bun, including top and bottom (1 1/2 oz)
Stuffing, bread, prepared	1/3 cup

Calories	Carb (g)	Fat (g)	Fiber (g)
78	15.1	0.5	0.6
127	17.0	5.8	0.5
75	14.0	1.0	1.0
75	14.0	1.0	1.0
80	15.2	1.0	2.1
71	13.6	1.1	1.1
85	19.0	1.0	4.0
91	20.1	1.1	5.5
95	20.4	1.1	4.5
83	15.5	1.1	1.9
80	16.0	0.5	1.0
80	15.0	1.0	1.0
67	12.4	0.9	0.6
70	12.0	1.0	2.0
69	12.9	1.2	1.9
75	16.0	0.0	2.0
70	10.0	2.0	1.0
113	18.5	3.0	1.0
67	13.1	0.5	0.8
60	10.6	0.9	0.5
61	10.8	1.1	0.6
75	12.0	2.0	0.0
82	15.7	1.2	0.6
82	16.7	0.4	0.7
85	14.3	2.1	0.9
75	16.0	0.0	2.0
100	20.0	1.0	5.0
117	14.3	5.7	1.9

continued

TABLE 8.1 *continued*

Food	Serving Size
Taco shells	2 medium (5" dia)
Tortilla, corn, ready to bake or fry	1 medium (6" dia)
Tortilla, flour, 10" across	1/3 tortilla
Tortilla, flour, 6" across	1 tortilla
Waffle, toaster-style	1 waffle (4" dia)
CEREALS	
All-Bran Cereal (Kellogg)	1/2 cup
Bran, oat, uncooked	1/4 cup
Bran,100% wheat, unprocessed	1/2 cup
Bran cereal (twigs, buds, or flakes)	1/2 cup
Cheerios	2/3 cup
Corn flakes	2/3 cup
Fiber One Bran Cereal (General Mills)	1/5 cup
Frosted Flakes Cereal (Kellogg)	1/5 cup
Granola	1/4 cup
Granola cereal, low-fat	1/4 cup
Grits, cooked	1/2 cup
Muesli	1/4 cup
Oatmeal, cooked	1/2 cup
Puffed rice cereal	1 1/2 cups
Puffed wheat cereal	1 1/2 cups
Rice krispies	3/4 cup
Shredded wheat, plain	1/2 cup
Sugar-coated cereal	1/2 cup
Unsweetened, ready-to-eat cereal	3/4 cup
Wheaties Cereal (General Mills)	3/4 cup
CRACKERS/SNACKS	
Animal crackers	8 crackers
Crackers, round butter-type	6 crackers
Crackers, saltines	6 crackers

Calories	Carb (g)	Fat (g)	Fiber (g)
124	16.6	6.0	2.0
52	10.7	0.7	1.5
72	11.9	1.8	0.7
112	0.5	2.8	1.1
96	14.6	3.3	0.5
81	22.9	1.0	9.9
58	15.6	1.7	3.6
63	18.7	1.2	12.4
80	21.0	0.5	6.0
83	16.6	1.4	2.0
76	18.1	0.2	0.7
59	24.3	0.8	14.4
76	18.6	0.1	0.7
125	19.0	4.9	1.3
86	18.0	1.1	1.1
70	16.0	0.0	0.0
74	15.1	1.1	1.5
73	12.6	1.2	2.0
80	18.4	0.2	0.3
66	13.8	0.4	1.7
77	17.4	0.3	0.1
83	20.3	0.3	2.8
70	15.0	0.5	1.0
85	18.0	0.0	1.0
80	18.2	0.7	2.3
89	14.8	2.8	0.2
90	11.0	4.6	0.3
77	12.8	2.0	0.5

continued

TABLE 8.1 *continued*

Food	Serving Size
Crackers, whole-wheat, baked	5 crackers
Crackers, whole-wheat, reduced-fat	5 triscuits
Crispbread	2–5 pieces (3/4 oz)
Graham crackers	3 crackers (2 1/2" square)
Matzoh crackers, plain	3/4 oz
Melba toast	4 pieces (3 3/4" x 1 3/4" x 1/8")
Nut and rice	10 crackers
Oyster crackers	20 crackers
Pita chips, baked	3/4 oz
Popcorn, microwave, 94% fat-free, popped	3 cups
Popcorn, microwave, with butter, popped	3 cups
Popcorn, popped, no salt or fat added	3 cups
Potato chips	3/4 oz
Potato chips, baked	3/4 oz
Potato chips, fat-free	3/4 oz
Pretzels, sticks or rings	3/4 oz
Rice cakes	2 cakes
Sandwich crackers, cheese-filled	3 sandwiches
Sandwich crackers, peanut butter	3 sandwiches
Tortilla chips	3/4 oz
Tortilla chips, fat-free	3/4 oz

STARCHY VEGETABLES

Food	Serving Size
Breadfruit	1/4 cup
Cassava, cooked	1/3 cup, diced
Corn on cob, cooked	1/2 large ear
Corn, canned, drained	1/2 cup
Corn, frozen, cooked	1/2 cup
Dasheen	1/3 cup
Hominy, canned, drained, rinsed	3/4 cup
Parsnips, fresh, cooked	1/2 cup

Calories	Carb (g)	Fat (g)	Fiber (g)
89	13.7	3.4	2.1
80	15.0	2.0	2.5
8	17.0	0.0	3.0
99	18.0	2.4	0.7
83	17.6	0.3	0.6
78	15.3	0.6	1.3
80	14.0	2.0	1.0
86	14.2	2.3	0.6
86	11.8	3.1	0.4
65	14.0	1.3	2.5
96	10.8	6.0	1.8
93	18.7	1.1	3.5
114	11.2	7.3	0.7
82	17.2	1.1	1.5
56	13.5	0.0	0.7
80	16.6	0.7	0.7
70	14.7	0.5	0.8
100	13.0	4.4	0.4
102	12.3	5.0	0.6
106	13.4	5.6	0.4
82	18.0	0.8	3.0
70	19.0	0.0	3.0
70	16.7	0.1	0.8
66	16.0	0.5	2.0
66	15.2	0.8	1.6
66	16.0	0.4	2.0
75	18.0	0.0	3.0
90	17.8	1.1	3.1
63	15.2	0.2	3.1

continued

TABLE 8.1 *continued*

Food	Serving Size
Pasta sauce, marinara, spaghetti sauce	1/2 cup
Peas, green	1/2 cup
Plantain, ripe, cooked	1/3 cup, slices
Potato, baked with skin	3 oz
Potato, fresh, mashed, made with milk	1/2 cup
Potato, white, peeled, cooked	3 oz
Potatoes, french-fried, frozen, oven-baked	1 cup
Pumpkin, canned, no-sugar-added	3/4 cup
Squash, winter, cooked	1 cup
Succotash (lima beans and corn), frozen	1/2 cup
Vegetables, mixed (corn, peas, carrots), frozen, cooked	1 cup
Vegetables, mixed (with pasta), frozen, cooked	1 cup
Yams, cooked	1/2 cup
BEANS/PEAS/LENTILS	
Beans, baked, no pork	1/3 cup
Beans, black, cooked	1/2 cup
Beans, kidney, cooked	1/2 cup
Beans, lima, canned, drained	1/2 cup
Beans, lima, frozen, cooked	1/2 cup
Beans, navy, cooked	1/2 cup
Beans, pinto, cooked	1/2 cup
Beans, white, cooked	1/2 cup
Chickpeas (garbanzo beans), cooked	1/2 cup
Lentils, cooked	1/2 cup
Peas, black-eyed (crowder), cooked	1/2 cup
Refried beans, canned	1/2 cup
Split peas, cooked	1/2 cup

Source: Adapted from *Choose Your Foods: Food Lists for Diabetes.* Academy of Nutrition and Dietetics and American Diabetes Association, 2014.

Calories	Carb (g)	Fat (g)	Fiber (g)
70	12.0	1.0	3.0
70	12.0	0.0	4.0
59	15.8	0.1	1.2
79	18.0	0.1	1.9
85	19.0	0.3	1.7
73	17.0	0.1	1.5
98	16.4	3.0	1.5
60	15.0	0.5	5.0
39	8.8	0.6	2.8
79	17.0	0.8	3.5
80	17.7	0.2	4.0
80	14.7	0.2	5.0
79	18.8	0.1	2.7
78	17.2	0.4	4.2
114	20.4	0.5	7.5
112	20.2	0.4	5.7
99	18.0	0.3	6.0
76	14.3	0.3	4.4
129	23.9	0.5	5.8
122	22.3	0.6	7.7
125	22.6	0.3	5.7
134	22.5	2.1	6.2
115	19.9	0.4	7.8
100	17.9	0.5	5.6
100	17.0	0.5	6.0
116	20.7	0.4	8.1

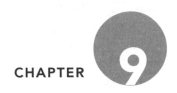

CHAPTER 9

Vegetables (Nonstarchy)

Foods in the Vegetable Group

This food group includes all fresh, frozen, and canned vegetables and vegetable juices. The vegetables in this food group are nonstarchy. You'll find starchy vegetables, such as corn, green peas, potatoes, and winter squash, in the starch group.

Vegetables are an extremely important part of your healthy eating plan. They are naturally packed with nutrition, yet are low in calories (if prepared healthfully). They provide lots of crunch for very few calories if they aren't fried or drowned in butter or salad dressing. As you strive to transition towards healthier eating habits, work towards having vegetables take up about half of your plate at lunch and dinner. And feel free to even work in vegetables at breakfast. Think vegetable juice, sautéed vegetables in an omelet or scrambled eggs, or slices of tomato and cucumber on a bagel.

The few calories that are in vegetables come from carbohydrate and a small amount of protein. Vegetables are good sources of fiber, vitamins, and minerals. Vary the vegetables you eat to get the variety of vitamins and minerals different vegetables offer.

The recommendations for vegetables from healthy eating guidelines are:

- 2 1/2 cups of vegetables each day.
- 1 1/2–2 cups of dark green vegetables each week.
- 4–6 cups of red and orange vegetables each week.

Nutrition Benefits of Vegetables

Different groups (or colors) of vegetables have different nutrition assets.

- **Dark green vegetables** include a variety of leafy greens, spinach, kale, broccoli, cabbage, brussels sprouts, and collards. They are often referred to as "nutrition powerhouses" because they are packed with fiber, beta-carotene (which the body converts to vitamin A), vitamins C and E, and minerals such as calcium, folate, potassium, and magnesium.

- **Red and orange vegetables** include carrots, red bell peppers, and tomatoes and are high in fiber, as well as other important nutrients. Carrots are a top source of beta-carotene, whereas bell peppers and tomatoes are rich in vitamin C. (Many of the other healthy orange vegetables, such as sweet potatoes and winter squash, are in the starch group.)

Nutrition studies have shown the benefits of eating vegetables. Together, vegetables and fruit have been shown to reduce the risk for and help manage type 2 diabetes, high blood pressure, and heart disease. They also protect against certain cancers, such as mouth, stomach, and colon cancer. Sound like a healthy bet?

Vegetables: How Much People Eat

People don't eat enough vegetables. Period. Do you? Most people eat only about half the recommended number of vegetable servings. That's not surprising with all of the on-the-go eating we do. Vegetables are just not plentiful in on-the-go venues and, yes, they do take a few extra minutes to prepare when eating at home.

Healthy Broccoli?

Vegetables are generally healthy, but if you douse your salads with blue cheese dressing, cover green beans with cream of mushroom soup, or order a fried onion or zucchini appetizer, then you've turned a healthy dish into something that is not! Here's how a healthy helping of broccoli quickly becomes unhealthy:

1 cup cooked broccoli = 44 calories
                                    0% calories from fat

  +

2 Tbsp cheese sauce = 36 calories, 4 g fat
                                    100% calories from fat

Now the broccoli has 80 calories, and 45% of those calories are from fat. That's still not a lot of calories, but there are flavorful ways to enjoy broccoli and other vegetables that don't pile on the calories. Take the Healthy Vegetable Challenge later in this chapter to learn more.

In addition to not eating enough vegetables in total, most people don't eat enough different kinds of vegetables, and neither do they take advantage of the most nutritious varieties. For example, many people choose light-colored iceberg lettuce for salads instead of the more nutritious dark-green spinach, arugula, red leaf lettuce, or romaine lettuce. Choosing from a variety of vegetables is important because it assures that you eat the wide array of beneficial nutrients you need. Variety also adds flavor and interest to your healthy eating plan.

Get to Know Yourself

If you want to change your eating habits, you need to take stock of your current eating habits. Ask yourself these questions about the vegetables you currently eat (or don't):

- How many servings of vegetables do I eat on average each day?
- What vegetables do I eat? Is it a short or long list?
- Do I eat some raw vegetables every day? With which meals?
- Do I buy vegetables packaged with a lot of added fat and sodium?
- Do I add fat and sodium to vegetables that I prepare?

How Many Vegetable Servings for You?

In chapter 6 you determined that a certain calorie range was the best for you to follow at the moment. Find that calorie range in Table 6.1, and then spot the number of vegetable servings you need to eat each day, either 4 or 5. This might seem like a lot of vegetables and may well be more than you currently eat. No problem! You'll learn easy ways to fit in more vegetables. (More is better when it comes to vegetables, and more vegetables will help you fill up on fewer calories.)

Get to Know Your Serving Sizes

Table 9.1 at the end of this chapter (starting on page 112) shows serving sizes for many vegetables you commonly eat, along with their calories, carbohydrate, and fiber content. Each vegetable serving, on average, contains about 5 grams of carbohydrate, 2 grams of protein, and 25 calories.

In general, one vegetable serving equals:

- 1 cup of raw vegetables.
- 1/2 cup of cooked vegetables.
- 1/2 cup of vegetable juice (see chapter 5 for more on juices).

It's important to eat the correct serving size, so you may want to weigh and measure your foods occasionally to make sure you're estimating correctly; however, if there's one place going a bit overboard won't hurt much, it's nonstarchy vegetables!

Sample Meal Plan

The sample meal plan below shows how you can fit 4 servings of vegetables into an eating plan with 1,400–1,600 calories a day. The vegetable servings are in bold for quick identification. Chapter 6 has sample meal plans and nutrition information for other calorie ranges.

ONE-DAY MEAL PLAN: **1,400–1,600 CALORIES**

BREAKFAST

1 whole-grain bagel thin (2 oz) with	2 starch
1 1/2 Tbsp light cream cheese	1 fat
3/4 cup blueberries with	1 fruit
1/3 cup fat-free plain yogurt	1/2 milk

LUNCH

Tuna salad made with	
3 oz tuna (1/2 cup), water-packed	3 oz protein
1 Tbsp light mayonnaise	1 fat
2 Tbsp diced celery	**1 vegetable**
1 Tbsp diced onions	
Tomato slices and lettuce leaves	1 free food
1 whole-wheat tortilla	2 starch
1 cup baby carrots	**1 vegetable**
1 cup fat-free milk	1 milk

DINNER

3 oz grilled salmon with	3 oz protein
lemon and herbs	free food
Stir-fried vegetables with	
1/4 cup onions, cooked	**2 vegetable**
1/2 cup snow peas, cooked	
1/2 cup red peppers, cooked	
2 tsp canola oil	2 fat
2/3 cup brown rice	2 starch

EVENING SNACK

Mix together:	
1/2 cup crushed canned pineapple	1 fruit
(packed in own juice)	
1/3 cup fat-free plain yogurt	1/2 milk
1/8 cup chopped pecans	2 fat

The Healthy Vegetable Challenge

Do you hide vegetables under cream sauce? Do you dunk raw vegetables in a sour cream– or mayonnaise–based dip? Do you buy frozen vegetables in cream or butter sauce? Do you buy canned vegetables, which are high in sodium? The Healthy Vegetable Challenge aims to find ways to prepare and eat vegetables with little to no added fat and sodium (see Table 9.2 for some examples). For example, instead of topping cooked vegetables with butter or margarine (either on your plate or a bowl of vegetables for the family),

TABLE 9.2	Higher-Fat Vegetable Options and Lower-Fat Alternatives		
Food	Serving	Calories	Fat (g)
Deep-fried zucchini, breaded	1/2 cup	279	16
Sautéed zucchini with broth and sherry	*1/2 cup*	*30*	*0*
Green bean casserole	1/2 cup	160	11
Green beans steamed with garlic and herbs	*1/2 cup*	*22*	*0*
Spinach soufflé	1/2 cup	110	9
Spinach, steamed	*1/2 cup*	*20*	*0*
Salad with 2 Tbsp regular blue cheese dressing	1 cup salad	191	16
Salad with 2 Tbsp fat-free blue cheese dressing	*1 cup salad*	*57*	*0*

Lower-fat alternatives are in italics.

squeeze some fresh lemon or lime juice on them. Or sprinkle cinnamon or nutmeg in the water when you microwave or boil carrots. These alternatives add flavor without adding fat.

It's also a healthy move to keep your vegetables' sodium content as low as possible. Vegetables are naturally very low in sodium, but the sodium creeps in when you use canned vegetables (unless they're the low-sodium kind), frozen vegetables with sauces and seasonings, or salads topped with salad dressing. Keep the sodium content of your vegetables low by using fresh vegetables or frozen or canned vegetables without added sauces.

Salad and Dressing Are Famous Food Pals

Perhaps the most famous vegetable-and-fat combo is salad with dressing. You select a nutrition-packed salad with dark greens, tomatoes, cucumbers, carrots, and more, which contains very few calories, mainly from carbohydrate. Then you pour on a couple of tablespoons of regular salad dressing, adding 150 calories of almost pure fat. It is challenging to keep your salads rich in nutrients and low in fat.

Watch out for those other high-fat salad toppings, too, such as cheese, bacon bits, or fried noodles. Dress up a salad with healthier toppings, such as olives, nuts, dried or chopped fruit, or seeds.

Salad Dressing Know-How

Your choice of salad dressings is wider than ever. In the supermarket, there are regular, reduced-fat, low-calorie, and fat-free salad dressings. Note that the terms "reduced-fat" and "fat-free" do not mean calorie-free. These dressings still contain calories. In fact, the fat-free dressings often contain more carbohydrate (to replace the fat), and many contain even more sodium. Check out the nutrition information for the different types of two of American's favorite dressings, Thousand Island and Italian, in Table 9.3.

Make It Homemade

One way to make sure your salad dressings are healthier, are lower in total fat, contain the healthiest fats, and are low in sodium is to make your own. Blend up a batch (it's easiest to just put all your ingredients in a blender), store it in a cruet or spray container, and bring it to the table instead of those bottled dressings. Make it with a healthy oil, one low in saturated fat. If you like the taste, use extra-virgin olive oil. If you like a lighter-tasting oil, use canola, sunflower, or soybean, or a combination. Choose from a wide variety of interesting vinegars, such as balsamic, raspberry, or red wine. Use a ratio of about two-thirds oil and one-third vinegar. The closer to half and half you can get, the fewer the calories. (A traditional vinaigrette is three-fourths oil, one-fourth vinegar.) Mustard can help emulsify (blend) the dressing. Season it with herbs and spices. Throw in some chopped or whole garlic cloves.

Tips to make your salad and dressing healthier pals:

• Don't add the dressing while you prepare the salad. Let the diner add the dressing when he or she eats it.

TABLE 9.3	Regular, Low-Calorie, and Fat-Free Thousand Island and Italian Salad Dressings			
Dressing	Calories (in 2 Tbsp)	Carbohydrate (g)	Fat (g)	Sodium (mg)
THOUSAND ISLAND				
Regular	118	5	11	276
Low-calorie	61	7	4	249
Fat-free	42	9	0.5	233
ITALIAN				
Regular	109	2	11	505
Low-calorie	56	2	6	398
Fat-free	20	4	0	430

- Use as little salad dressing as you can. (Hint: If you always find dressing at the bottom of your salad, that's proof you can use less.)

- Use the fork-and-dip technique. Serve the dressing on the side, and lightly dip a forkful of salad into the dressing.

- If you use a creamy dressing, dilute it with a few drizzles of your preferred vinegar or lemon.

- In fast-food restaurants, don't use the whole packet, which amounts to 1/4 cup (4 tablespoons). Drizzle on some dressing, mix up your salad, and see if you have enough.

Eat More Vegetables

An easy way to eat more vegetables is to eat them raw: a few spears of broccoli or cauliflower, a handful of cherry or grape tomatoes, a handful of baby carrots, or sticks of zucchini or yellow squash. If you eat raw vegetables, you retain the vitamins and minerals that are lost when you cook them. Stock your refrigerator with a ready-to-go supply of vegetables and have a handful for lunch, dinner, or a snack. Make enough salad at one time to last a few days, or chop and store the salad extras: peppers, red cabbage, cucumbers, carrots, onions, and the like. Store them in an airtight plastic container.

If you do not like some vegetables raw, but you will eat them cooked and chilled, blanch a bunch of green beans, a head of broccoli or cauliflower, or a handful of snow peas. Stash them in a plastic container in the refrigerator so that they are ready to eat. How do you blanch vegetables? Boil a small amount of water and steam the vegetables for 2–3 minutes. Vegetables should be slightly soft but still crisp. Remove the pot from the stove or microwave and place the vegetables in ice water to stop the cooking process. You can also cook vegetables in the microwave and then douse them in ice water to stop the cooking process.

Tips for Buying, Preparing, and Eating More Vegetables

- Vary your vegetables. The greater the variety, the greater the mix of vitamins, minerals, and other nutrients you will eat.

- Take advantage of all the ready-to-eat or easy-to-fix vegetables in the supermarket: salad in bags or boxes, baby carrots, grape and cherry tomatoes, precut celery and carrot sticks, sliced mushrooms, and bags of precut vegetable medleys ready to steam.

- Keep a bag of precut carrots around. Have a handful as a snack, pack them with lunch, add them to stew, or microwave them for a quick dish.

- Have on hand frozen and low-sodium canned vegetables to assure you'll always have vegetables ready to eat.

- So many salad greens are available today that it's easy to have a variety of several greens in your salads—romaine, mixed field greens, arugula, or spinach. Dice in some red cabbage for color and nutrition. If you buy bags or boxes of greens, choose ones that combine several types.

- Don't buy vegetables packed in butter or flavored sauces.

- Make double and triple portions. Eat a serving one day, and have another one ready to go for the next.

- Blanch (quickly cook and chill) a head of broccoli or cauliflower, break it into pieces, place them in a plastic container, and have a ready supply for the week, hot or cold.

- Microwave or sauté onions, peppers, and mushrooms to add more vegetables to a tomato sauce or top a frozen pizza.

- Enjoy baby carrots, celery sticks, and slices of red pepper dipped in a yogurt-based dip or reduced-calorie creamy salad dressing for a low-calorie snack.

- Make a big salad to last a few days; store it in a plastic container.

- Remember, almost anything healthy can top a salad: green peas, garbanzo beans, green beans, bulgur, quinoa, brown rice, raisins, pineapple, dried apricots, or mandarin oranges. The list can go on and on!

- Add vegetables to sandwiches—not just lettuce and sliced tomato. Try alfalfa sprouts or slices of red onion, cucumbers, yellow squash, zucchini, or red peppers. Use avocado slices instead of mayonnaise to moisten the bread.

- Add vegetables to an omelet or scrambled eggs. Sauté onions, peppers, mushrooms, and tomatoes in a healthy oil or a bit of water or broth to minimize calories, and add some fresh herbs.

- In a tomato sauce, cut the amount of meat you use in half and add more vegetables: onions, peppers, mushrooms, eggplant, zucchini, or others.

- Use puréed cooked vegetables such as potatoes to thicken stews, soups, and gravies. These add flavor, nutrients, and texture.

- Keep cans of vegetable juice on hand to grab for an on-the-run, take-the-edge-off-your-appetite snack, to use in cooking, or to enjoy with a meal.

| TABLE 9.1 | Serving Sizes, Calories, and Nutrients for Vegetables |

Food	Serving Size
VEGETABLES	
Amaranth leaves (Chinese spinach), cooked	1/2 cup
Artichoke hearts, canned, drained	1 artichoke
Artichoke, cooked	1/2 artichoke
Asparagus, frozen, cooked	1/2 cup
Baby corn, cocktail-type, canned, drained	1/2 cup
Bamboo shoots, canned, drained	1/2 cup
Bean sprouts, fresh, cooked	1/2 cup
Beans, canned, drained (green, wax)	1/2 cup
Beans, green, fresh, cooked	1/2 cup
Beans, Italian	1/2 cup
Beans, yard-long	1/2 cup
Beets, canned, drained	1/2 cup
Bitter melon gourd (Asian, balsam), cooked	1/2 cup (1/2" pieces)
Bok choy (Chinese white cabbage or pak-choy)	1 cup, shredded
Borscht (beet soup)	1/2 cup
Broccoli, fresh, cooked	1/2 cup
Brussels sprouts, frozen, cooked	1/2 cup
Cabbage, fresh, cooked	1/2 cup
Carrots, fresh, cooked	1/2 cup
Carrots, fresh, raw	1 cup, strips or sticks
Cauliflower, fresh, raw	1 cup
Cauliflower, frozen, cooked	1/2 cup
Celery, fresh, raw	1 cup, strips
Chard, Swiss, cooked	1/2 cup
Chayote squash (mirliton, sayote), cooked	1/2 cup
Coleslaw mix	1 cup
Collard greens, fresh, cooked	1/2 cup
Cucumber, with peel	1 cup
Daikon	1/2 cup
Eggplant, fresh, cooked	1/2 cup (1" cubes)

Calories	Carb (g)	Fiber (g)
14	2.7	1.2
15	3.0	0.5
30	7.3	0.5
25	4.4	1.4
20	5.0	2.0
12	2.1	0.9
13	2.6	0.5
14	3.1	1.3
22	4.9	2.0
20	5.0	2.0
25	5.0	2.0
26	6.1	1.4
12	2.7	1.2
9	1.5	0.7
39	4.1	0.9
22	4.0	2.3
33	6.5	3.3
17	3.3	1.7
35	8.2	2.6
50	11.7	3.7
25	5.2	2.5
17	3.4	2.4
17	3.7	1.7
18	3.6	1.8
19	4.1	2.2
17	3.3	1.5
26	5.8	2.7
16	3.8	0.5
10	3.0	1.0
17	4.3	1.2

continued

TABLE 9.1 *continued*

Food	Serving Size
Fennel	1/2 cup
Gourd (bitter, bottle)	1/2 cup
Green (spring) onions	1 cup
Greens, dandelion	1/2 cup
Greens, purslane	1/2 cup
Hearts of palm, canned, not drained	1/2 cup
Jicama (yambean, singkamas), cooked	1/2 cup, cubes
Kale, fresh, cooked	1/2 cup
Kohlrabi, fresh, cooked	1/2 cup
Leeks, fresh, cooked	1/2 cup
Luffa (Chinese okra), angled, cooked	1/2 cup
Mixed vegetables (no corn, peas, pasta)	1/2 cup
Mung bean sprouts, seed attached, cooked	1/2 cup
Mushrooms, fresh	1 cup
Mustard greens, fresh, cooked	1/2 cup
Okra, frozen, cooked	1/2 cup
Onions, fresh	1 cup
Onions, fresh, cooked	1/2 cup
Oriental radish (daikon, labanos), raw	1 cup
Pea pods (snow peas), fresh, cooked	1/2 cup
Peas, sugar snap, frozen, uncooked	1/2 cup
Pepper, green bell, raw	1 cup, slices
Pepper, red, fresh, cooked	1/2 cup
Peppers, hot chile, green, canned	1/2 cup
Radishes	1 cup
Rutabaga, fresh, cooked	1/2 cup, cubes
Sauerkraut, canned, rinsed, drained	1/2 cup
Soybean sprouts, seed attached, cooked	1/2 cup
Spinach, canned, drained	1/2 cup
Squash, summer, fresh, cooked	1/2 cup

Calories	Carb (g)	Fiber (g)
25	6.0	3.0
10	3.0	1.0
32	7.3	2.6
15	3.0	2.0
10	2.0	0.0
20	3.4	1.8
30	6.9	3.1
18	3.7	1.3
24	5.5	0.9
16	4.0	0.5
20	4.0	2.0
20	3.3	1.3
13	2.6	0.5
15	2.3	0.7
10	1.5	1.4
34	5.3	2.6
67	16.2	2.2
46	10.7	1.5
21	4.8	1.9
34	5.6	2.2
30	5.2	1.9
18	4.3	1.6
19	4.6	0.8
25	3.3	3.3
20	4.2	1.9
33	7.4	1.5
23	5.1	3.0
38	3.1	0.4
25	3.6	2.6
18	3.9	1.3

continued

TABLE 9.1 *continued*	
Food	**Serving Size**
Squash, summer, raw	1 cup
Tomato juice	1/2 cup
Tomato sauce	1/2 cup
Tomato, raw	1 cup
Tomatoes, canned, regular	1/2 cup
Turnip greens, fresh, cooked	1/2 cup
Turnips, fresh, cooked	1/2 cup, diced
Vegetable juice	1/2 cup
Water chestnuts, canned, drained	1/2 cup
Yard-long beans, fresh, cooked	1/2 cup, slices
Zucchini, fresh, cooked	1/2 cup, slices
Zucchini, raw	1 cup, slices

Source: Adapted from *Choose Your Foods: Food Lists for Diabetes.* Academy of Nutrition and Dietetics and American Diabetes Association, 2014.

Calories	Carb (g)	Fiber (g)
18	3.8	1.2
21	5.2	0.5
37	8.8	1.7
32	7.1	2.2
24	5.5	1.3
14	3.1	2.5
17	3.9	1.6
25	5.5	0.5
40	8.9	2.7
24	4.8	1.9
14	3.5	1.3
18	3.8	1.2

CHAPTER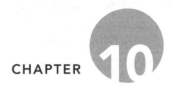

Fruits

Foods in the Fruit Group

The fruit group includes all fresh, frozen, canned, and dried fruits and fruit juices. Fruits are an important part of your healthy eating plan because they're naturally packed with vitamins, minerals, and fiber. Fruits have a moderate amount of calories, mainly from carbohydrate, and no calories from fat. Fruits can satisfy your sweet tooth.

Fruits are excellent sources of vitamins A and C and minerals such as potassium, magnesium, folate, and copper. They naturally contain no fat, very little sodium, and no cholesterol. Most fruits provide some fiber, but how much depends on the form of the fruit you eat as well as the type. For example, a fresh apple provides more fiber than applesauce, apple juice has no fiber, and berries contain more fiber than an apple.

When you vary the fruits you eat, you get the variety of vitamins and minerals they offer. Nutrition studies have shown numerous benefits of eating a sufficient amount of fruit each day. These studies usually also consider the benefits of eating more vegetables, too. Together, eating more fruits and vegetables has been shown to reduce the risk for and to help manage prediabetes, type 2 diabetes, high blood pressure, and heart disease. They can assist with weight control and can protect against certain cancers, such as mouth, stomach, and colon cancer.

Fruits Offer a Variety of Nutrients

- Berries offer a good source of vitamin C and fiber.

- Citrus fruits, kiwi, guava, papaya, and cantaloupe are well known for their high vitamin C content.

- Orange fruits, such as mango, apricot, red or pink grapefruit, and cantaloupe, are sources of vitamin A.

- Oranges, bananas, dried fruits, cantaloupe, and honeydew are sources of potassium.

- Oranges and orange juice can also tout their superior folate (folic acid) content.

How Much Fruit People Eat

When it comes to eating enough fruit, most people would get an F. We eat about half of the recommended 2 1/2 cups we need each day. In general, young children and older adults eat the most fruit. This occurs for a few reasons. Once you leave your kitchen, it's hard to find fruit, and if you do, it's so expensive you may resist the purchase. Fruit is not plentiful in restaurants; the situation is even worse than with vegetables. Fortunately, a great variety of fruits is available in the supermarket year-round and more restaurants, particularly fast-food and sandwich shops, now have more fruit on their menus. Similar to vegetables, people don't vary the fruits they eat enough—most people limit their selection to apples, oranges, and bananas.

Get to Know Yourself

If you want to change your eating habits, you need to assess your current eating habits. Ask yourself these questions about the fruits you eat (or don't eat):

- How many servings of fruit do I eat on average each day? Is this enough or too much?

- When during the day do I usually eat fruit? At meals, which ones? For snacks, which ones?

- What fruits do I eat? Is it a narrow or wide selection?

- What forms of fruits do I buy?

- Do I buy and drink a lot of fruit juice? What's a usual serving at home or in restaurants?

- Do I think fruit causes problems with my blood glucose levels?

Best Form of Fruit to Eat

Fresh fruit is your best bet to maximize fiber from fruit. When fresh fruit isn't available or affordable, fruit that is canned or packaged with no sugar added or sweetened with a no-calorie sweetener is a healthy alternative; unsweetened applesauce is one example. Dried fruits such as raisins, apricots, dried apples, and dates are excellent sources of nutrition. They are not as perishable as fresh fruit and make a good option for carry-along snacks. However, portion control matters. They're concentrated sources of carbohydrate, and it's easy to eat too much of them.

Drink as little fruit juice as possible. While it offers good nutrition, especially if it's fortified with extra nutrition such as vitamin D and calcium, fruit juice contains nearly no fiber, even orange juice with pulp. Plus, if you're quenching your thirst, it can be challenging to drink only the small amount in one serving (about 1/2 cup, which is 4 ounces). A typical container of juice from a convenience store is 12–16 ounces—that's 3 to 4 fruit servings. See chapter 15 for more on fruit juices and smoothies.

How Many Servings of Fruit for You?

In chapter 6, you determined which calorie range was the best for you to follow. Find that calorie range in Table 6.1, and then spot the number of servings of fruit to eat each day. It's somewhere between 2 and 4. This might seem like a lot of fruit to eat based on your current eating habits. Keep in mind that people with diabetes can control their blood glucose while they enjoy fruit and should eat fruit for its nutrition and health benefits.

Get to Know Your Serving Sizes

Table 10.1 at the end of this chapter (starting on page 128) shows serving sizes for many fruits you commonly eat, along with their calories, carbohydrate, and fiber. Each fruit serving, on average, contains about 15 grams of carbohydrates and 60 calories.

In general, one fruit serving equals:

- 1 small, medium, or half a large piece of fruit (servings vary).
- 1/2 cup of canned fruit packed with no sugar added.
- 1/2 cup of unsweetened fruit juice.
- 1/4 cup of dried fruit.

Get familiar with the sizes and servings of the fruits you eat. It's a good idea to weigh and measure them as you increase your awareness of serving sizes. Then repeat this "calibration" regularly. It's very easy to eat larger servings than you need.

Sample Meal Plan

The sample meal plan below gives you an idea of how to fit 2 servings of fruits into an eating plan with 1,400–1,600 calories a day. You'll see that the fruit servings are in bold for quick identification. Chapter 6 provides sample meal plans and nutrition information for other calorie ranges.

ONE-DAY MEAL PLAN: 1,400–1,600 CALORIES

BREAKFAST

1 whole-grain bagel thin (2 oz) with	2 starch
1 1/2 Tbsp light cream cheese	1 fat
3/4 cup blueberries with	**1 fruit**
1/3 cup fat-free plain yogurt	1/2 milk

LUNCH

Tuna salad made with	
3 oz tuna (1/2 cup), water-packed	3 oz protein
1 Tbsp light mayonnaise	1 fat
2 Tbsp diced celery	1 vegetable
1 Tbsp diced onions	
Tomato slices and lettuce leaves	1 free food
1 whole-wheat tortilla	2 starch
1 cup baby carrots	1 vegetable
1 cup fat-free milk	1 milk

DINNER

3 oz grilled salmon with	3 oz protein
lemon and herbs	free food
Stir-fried vegetables with	
1/4 cup onions, cooked	2 vegetable
1/2 cup snow peas, cooked	
1/2 cup red peppers, cooked	
2 tsp canola oil	2 fat
2/3 cup brown rice	2 starch

EVENING SNACK

Mix together:

1/2 cup crushed canned pineapple	**1 fruit**
(packed in own juice)	
1/3 cup fat-free plain yogurt	1/2 milk
1/8 cup chopped pecans	2 fat

Fruit and Blood Glucose Control

In general, fruit does not raise blood glucose faster than other sources of carbohydrate. The challenge is to determine how fruit in general and specific fruits affect your blood glucose. Does eating fruit in the morning make it more difficult for you to keep your blood glucose on target throughout the day? Does one particular kind or form of fruit raise your blood glucose higher than others? Does a piece of fruit as an afternoon snack give you just enough carbohydrate to last until dinner? The answers to these questions need to dovetail with whether you take enough and the right types of blood glucose–lowering medication. Yes, it can get complex, but don't avoid fruit, or other healthy foods, as a way to control your blood glucose. It's simply too healthy!

The effect of fruit on your blood glucose levels depends on many factors:

- The form of the fruit—is it juice that you gulp in seconds or a piece of fresh fruit that takes a few minutes to eat?

- Whether you eat the fruit as part of a meal, at the end of the meal, or by itself as a snack.

- The glycemic index (GI) or glycemic load of the fruit (see chapter 3).

Determine the fruit that is best for you to eat after you consider your nutrition and blood glucose goals. Figure out whether it's best to have fruit at meals or snacks. Eat the fruit, either alone or with other foods as a meal or snack, and check your blood glucose level about 1–2 hours after you eat it. Use your blood glucose monitoring results to answer your questions about fruit.

Dress Fruit Up for Dessert

Fruit makes a great dessert, from apple cobbler to blueberry pie. The problem is that many calories and grams of fat and carbohydrate are added before the dessert enters your mouth. Table 10.2 shows just a few examples of how fruit can be a healthy low-calorie dessert or a less healthy high-calorie one. Search for ways to prepare fruits that will satisfy your sweet tooth but not get in the way of your nutrition goals.

Start with these:

- Baked apples, lower-calorie apple cobbler, or applesauce.

- Banana bread or frozen bananas rolled in cocoa or chopped nuts.

- Sliced bananas or canned peaches or pears in fat-free, sugar-free pudding mix.

- Frozen (no-sugar-added) blueberries or strawberries on frozen yogurt or topped with plain yogurt.

- Frozen (no-sugar-added) blueberries or strawberries on angel food cake.

- Sliced fresh fruit or fruit kabobs dipped in fruited yogurt or other low-calorie dip.

Tips for Buying, Preparing, and Eating More Fruit

- Take advantage of the precut, ready-to-eat fruit available in today's supermarkets. They make it easy to have fruit anytime.
- Add berries to cereal, plain yogurt, or light sour cream or use them to top pancakes, waffles, ice cream, or frozen yogurt.
- Add slices of banana or peaches to cold cereal.
- Add raisins, pieces of dried apricot, or chopped apple when cooking hot cereal.
- Keep a plastic container full of cut-up fruit, so you can have some at breakfast or for a snack topped with fat-free plain or fruited yogurt (for more calcium).
- Take one or two pieces of fruit from home each day (if you spend most of the day away from home) to eat with lunch, as an afternoon snack, or on your way home to take the edge off your hunger.
- Keep dried fruit, raisins, figs, apricots, peaches, or pears around for a snack, for fuel on long hikes or bike rides, or to stash in your desk or locker. (Watch your serving sizes.)
- Have canned or jarred fruit with no sugar added at the ready in the pantry: applesauce, peaches, pears, and pineapple are just a start.
- Keep frozen fruit with no added sugar in your freezer. Blend it into a breakfast shake or smoothie, or use as a topping for ice cream or frozen yogurt.
- Put fruit into entrées: pineapple in stir-fry or on pizza, fresh or dried cranberries or peaches in chicken dishes, or apricots or apples in pork dishes.
- Serve fruit with the main course: applesauce with pork chops or roast, pineapple with ham, or homemade cranberry sauce with chicken.

TABLE 10.2 High-Calorie and Low-Calorie Dessert Choices

Food	Serving	Calories	Fat (g)
Apple crisp	1 cup	194	8
Apple (medium), peeled and baked with low-calorie sweetener and cinnamon	*1*	*73*	*0*
Banana cream pie	1 piece	398	20
Banana bread	*1 slice*	*120*	*5*
Strawberry ice cream	1 cup	254	11
Strawberries (frozen) on 1 piece angel food cake	*1/2 cup*	*194*	*0*

Healthier alternatives are in italics.

TABLE 10.1	Serving Sizes, Calories, and Nutrients for Fruits
Food	**Serving Size**
FRESH/CANNED/DRIED FRUITS	
Apple, with peel	1 small (4 oz)
Apples, dried	4 rings
Applesauce, unsweetened	1/2 cup
Apricots, canned, juice pack	1/2 cup, halves
Apricots, dried	8 halves
Apricots, fresh	4 apricots
Banana, fresh	1 extra small (<6" long)
Blackberries, fresh	3/4 cup
Blueberries, dried	2 Tbsp
Blueberries, fresh	3/4 cup
Cantaloupe melon, fresh	1 cup
Cherries, canned, juice pack, sweet	1/2 cup
Cherries, dried	2 Tbsp
Cherries, sweet, fresh	12 cherries
Cranberries, dried	2 Tbsp
Dates	3 dates
Figs, dried	1 1/2 figs
Figs, fresh	2 medium (2 1/4" dia)
Fruit cocktail, canned, juice pack	1/2 cup
Grapefruit sections, canned	3/4 cup
Grapefruit, fresh	1/2 grapefruit
Grapes, fresh, seedless, small	17 grapes
Guavas	2 small (2 1/2 oz total)
Honeydew melon, fresh	1 cup, diced
Kiwi	1/2 cup, slices
Loquat	3/4 cup, cubes
Mandarin oranges, canned, juice pack	3/4 cup
Mango, fresh	1/2 mango, small
Nectarine, fresh	1 small (5 oz)
Orange, fresh	1 orange

Calories	Carb (g)	Fiber (g)
54	14.4	2.5
63	17.1	2.3
52	13.8	1.5
59	15.1	2.0
67	17.5	2.0
67	15.6	3.4
72	18.5	2.1
56	13.8	5.7
69	16.0	1.0
62	15.8	2.6
56	13.4	1.3
68	17.3	1.9
66	16.0	1.0
59	13.6	1.9
47	12.5	0.9
69	18.5	1.9
71	18.2	2.8
74	19.2	3.3
60	14.0	1.0
69	17.2	0.7
53	13.4	1.8
60	15.1	0.8
75	16.0	6.0
61	15.5	1.4
55	13.0	3.0
55	14.0	2.0
69	17.9	1.3
68	17.7	1.9
60	14.3	2.3
62	15.4	3.1

continued

TABLE 10.1 *continued*

Food	Serving Size
Papaya, fresh	1 cup, cubes
Peach, fresh	1 medium
Peaches, canned, juice pack	1/2 cup
Pear, fresh	1/2 large (approx 2 per lb)
Pears, canned, juice pack	1/2 cup
Pineapple, canned, juice pack	1/2 cup
Pineapple, fresh	3/4 cup
Plantain, extra-ripe (black), raw	1/4 plantain (2 1/4 oz)
Plums, fresh	2 plums (2 1/8" dia)
Plums, canned, juice pack	1/2 cup
Plums, dried (prunes)	3 prunes
Pomegranate seeds (arils)	1/2 cup
Raisins, dark, seedless	2 Tbsp
Raspberries, fresh	1 cup
Strawberries, fresh	1 1/4 cups
Tangerines, fresh	2 small
Watermelon, fresh	1 1/4 cups
FRUIT JUICES	
Apple juice or cider, canned or bottled	1/2 cup
Fruit juice blends, 100% juice	1/3 cup
Grape juice	1/3 cup
Grapefruit juice, canned	1/2 cup
Orange juice, fresh	1/2 cup
Pineapple juice, canned	1/2 cup
Pomegranate juice	1/2 cup
Prune juice, bottled	1/3 cup

Source: Adapted from *Choose Your Foods: Food Lists for Diabetes.* Academy of Nutrition and Dietetics and American Diabetes Association, 2014.

Calories	Carb (g)	Fiber (g)
55	13.7	2.5
57	14.0	1.9
55	14.3	1.6
61	16.2	3.2
62	16.0	2.0
74	19.5	1.0
56	14.7	1.6
50	13.0	1.0
61	15.1	1.8
73	19.1	1.3
60	15.6	1.8
70	16.0	1.0
54	14.2	0.7
60	14.2	8.4
57	13.3	4.4
81	20.3	2.7
57	14.3	0.8
58	14.5	0.1
50	11.6	0.1
50	12.5	0.1
47	11.1	0.1
56	12.9	0.2
70	17.2	0.3
65	16.0	0.0
59	14.7	0.9

CHAPTER 11

Milks and Yogurts

What's Ahead?

→ Foods included in this food group.

→ The nutrition assets of milk (all types) and yogurt.

→ Healthy eating goals for milk and yogurt.

→ How to assess the servings of milk and yogurt you consume now.

→ The ideal number of servings of milk and yogurt for you.

→ The dairy, calcium, and osteoporosis connection.

→ Tips to help you buy, prepare, and consume more milk and yogurt.

→ Serving sizes and nutrition numbers for milks and yogurts.

Foods in the Milks and Yogurts Group

This group includes all types of cow's milk and other types of milk, like soy milk and rice milk. You'll find unsweetened nut milks such as almond and coconut milk in the fat food group due to their nutrition makeup. Yogurts, including regular and Greek yogurt, plain, with fruit, flavored, or unflavored, are in this group. The variety of milks and yogurts available today is wider than ever.

Dairy products that contain little to no calcium, such as cream cheese, cream, and butter, are generally found in the fat group. You'll find cheese in the protein group. Other than being a great source of calcium, cheese has more in common nutritionally with meats because it contains mainly protein and fat.

Fat-free milks and fat-free plain yogurts are healthy packages of carbohydrate and protein. You may not think about milk and yogurt as sources of carbohydrate, but an 8-ounce glass of milk contains nearly as much carbohydrate as a slice of bread or 1/3 cup of pasta. An 8-ounce glass of flavored, low-fat rice milk contains nearly 30 grams of carbohydrate. A serving of cow's milk, soy milk, or yogurt contains about as much protein as one ounce of meat. Rice milk contains less protein, whereas Greek yogurt contains a bit more. If you use fat-free milks and yogurts, they contain nearly no fat, so there's no saturated fat, trans fat, or cholesterol.

Milk and yogurt contain no fiber, although some brands of yogurt now contain added fiber. (A common fiber used is inulin.) They're excellent sources of many vitamins and minerals, including calcium, vitamin D (when fortified), and potassium, which are three nutrients most people don't eat enough of. You're much more likely to get adequate amounts of these essential nutrients if you consume 3 servings a day from this food group.

Host of Health Benefits

Healthy bones and the prevention of osteoporosis are the well-known benefits of getting enough calcium. Over the last few years, even more health benefits have been attributed to dairy foods. Sufficient intake of low-fat and fat-free dairy foods has been linked to reduced risk of cardiovascular disease and better control of blood pressure.

Osteoporosis

More than 50 million people in America have either osteoporosis (9 million) or low bone mass (osteopenia) (43 million), which places them at increased risk for broken bones. Hip fractures are the most common bone fractures that people experience. Osteopenia and osteoporosis are more common in women and older adults. In addition, research is showing that people with type 1 diabetes, particularly those diagnosed at a young age, and people with type 2 diabetes, particularly those who are overweight, may be more likely to have osteopenia or osteoporosis and experience bone fractures. Other long-term diabetes complications such as vision problems and nerve damage may add to this increased risk of falls and fractures.

Tips to Prevent Osteoporosis

The best way to prevent osteoporosis is to get enough calcium throughout your life, so speak to your children and grandchildren about eating sufficient amounts of milk and yogurt.

- Get enough calcium from milks, yogurts, and other high-calcium foods.

- Take a calcium supplement with extra vitamin D to maximize calcium absorption if you don't get enough calcium from your foods. (Most people don't.) Talk to your health-care provider about whether you need a calcium supplement and, if so, which one is best for you. Today they come in a number of different forms.

- Do weight-bearing activities—walk, jog, dance, garden, or lift light weights—a few times a week. Weight-bearing exercise helps you maintain your bone and muscle mass, especially as you age.

Blood Pressure

High blood pressure, also referred to as hypertension, is a major risk factor for heart disease and stroke. It's common among older adults and especially common among people with diabetes. Several studies have shown that consuming enough low-fat dairy foods, along with fruits and vegetables, can help lower blood pressure. Read about more about sodium, potassium, and blood pressure control and the DASH (Dietary Approaches to Stop Hypertension) study and diet in chapter 4.

Milks and Yogurts: How Americans Eat

People consume about half of the recommended amount of milk and yogurt and are not getting enough calcium, potassium, and other vital nutrients in their diets. Milk is often missing from meals, particularly at restaurants. Consumption of cereal, milk's best friend, is also on the decline, which translates to another lost opportunity to consume milk. Fortunately, yogurt is growing in popularity, particularly with younger adults, although the use of rice, soy, and other milks remains relatively small.

Get to Know Yourself

If you want to change your eating habits, you need to assess your current eating habits. Ask yourself these questions about the milks and yogurts group:

- How many servings of milk or yogurt do I consume on an average day? Is this enough or too much?

- Do I correctly estimate the servings of milk or yogurt I eat?

- What type of milk and yogurt do I buy: fat-free, 2%, full-fat, almond (this is in the fat food group), rice, soy, fruited, flavored, or unflavored?

- Do I get the amount of calcium and potassium I need each day to meet my nutritional needs?

- Am I at risk for osteopenia or osteoporosis?

- Do I buy calcium-fortified foods when possible, or add milk or yogurt to my dishes so I get more calcium?

How Many Servings of Milk and Yogurt for You?

In chapter 6, you determined that a certain calorie range was the best for you to follow at the moment. Find that calorie range in Table 6.1. Then spot the number of servings of milk and yogurt to consume each day. You'll see it's 2 servings a day for all meal plans. However, if you can sneak in a third serving without going overboard on calories, you'll more often meet your calcium goals. In this chapter, you'll learn easy ways to consume more milk and yogurt.

Get to Know Your Serving Sizes

Table 11.1 at the end of the chapter (starting on page 144) shows serving sizes for the milks and yogurts in this food group, along with their calories, carbohydrate, protein, and fat content. Each serving contains about 12 grams of carbohydrate and 8 grams of protein. The amount of calories in each serving depends on the amount of fat in it. Fat-free products contain about 80–100 calories, whereas products that contain more fat, like whole milk, contain 8 grams of fat and 150 calories per serving.

In general, one serving equals:

- 1 cup (8 ounces) of any type of milk (other than almond milk).

- 2/3–1 cup (6–8 ounces) of various types of yogurt.

Portions are important. It's good to occasionally measure the amount of milk and yogurt you consume to make sure your portions are correct. Another portion-control tip: drink and eat these foods from the same cup or bowl as often as possible.

Sample Meal Plan

The sample meal plan below gives you an idea of how to fit 2 servings of milk and yogurt into an eating plan with 1,400–1,600 calories a day. You'll see that the milk and yogurt servings are in bold for quick identification. Chapter 6 provides sample meal plans and nutrition information for the other calorie ranges.

ONE-DAY MEAL PLAN: **1,400–1,600 CALORIES**

BREAKFAST

1 whole-grain bagel thin (2 oz) with	2 starch
1 1/2 Tbsp light cream cheese	1 fat
3/4 cup blueberries with	1 fruit
1/3 cup fat-free plain yogurt	**1/2 milk**

LUNCH

Tuna salad made with	
3 oz tuna (1/2 cup), water-packed	3 oz protein
1 Tbsp light mayonnaise	1 fat
2 Tbsp diced celery	1 vegetable
1 Tbsp diced onions	
Tomato slices and lettuce leaves	1 free food
1 whole-wheat tortilla	2 starch
1 cup baby carrots	1 vegetable
1 cup fat-free milk	**1 milk**

DINNER

3 oz grilled salmon with	3 oz protein
lemon and herbs	free food
Stir-fried vegetables with	

1/4 cup onions, cooked	2 vegetable
1/2 cup snow peas, cooked	
1/2 cup red peppers, cooked	
2 tsp canola oil	2 fat
2/3 cup brown rice	2 starch

EVENING SNACK

Mix together:

1/2 cup crushed canned pineapple (packed in own juice)	1 fruit
1/3 cup fat-free plain yogurt	**1/2 milk**
1/8 cup chopped pecans	2 fat

Calcium: How Much and from Which Foods?

Table 11.2 shows the current recommendations for calcium for the general public across all age ranges. People with diabetes can follow these recommendations, too. The best food sources of calcium are dairy products—milk, yogurt, and cheese. Other nondairy sources of calcium are dark green leafy vegetables (such as broccoli, kale, and collards), sardines, and canned salmon.

Today, you can buy more products that are calcium-fortified, like soy, rice, and almond milk; fruit juices, such as orange, grapefruit, and apple juice; and hot and cold cereals. Table 5.3 on page 52 is a list of the top 10 sources of calcium.

Note that the sample meal plan in this chapter contains nearly 900 mg of calcium, still under the goal for most adults but much higher than what most people achieve each day. In the sample meal plan, you'd reach 1,000 milligrams easily if you substituted canned salmon for tuna fish at lunch, mixed a handful of spinach or other dark green leafy vegetables into your stir-fried vegetables at dinner, used calcium-fortified fat-free milk, or took a multivitamin that contains at least 200 mg of calcium (the usual amount).

TABLE 11.2	Daily Calcium Recommendations
Age Ranges	**Calcium Recommendation (mg)**
Girls and boys: ages 1–3	700
Girls and boys: ages 4–8	1,000
Girls and boys: ages 9–18	1,300
Women and men: ages 19–50	1,000
Women: age 51 and older	1,200
Women: pregnant or breast-feeding, over age 18	1,000
Men: age 51 and older	1,000

A Maze of Milks and Yogurts

Supermarket shelves today stock fat-free and whole milk, soy milk, lactose-free milk, and more. As often as you can, choose a type of fat-free milk to get all the nutrients you need.

Some people think they save lots of calories and trim fat grams when they move from whole milk to 2% milk, but that's not so. Whole milk contains only 3 1/2% fat and about 150 calories per 8 ounces, whereas 2% has about 120 calories. That's not a big difference. However, with a couple of cups of milk a day, these calories can add up. Fat-free milk has about 90 calories per 8 ounces. If you drink soy or rice milk, choose a fat-free, calcium-fortified, unflavored type; however, you still won't get some of the nutrients cow's milk offers.

If you are lactose intolerant, drink lactose-free milk if you tolerate it and like it. Buy calcium-fortified lactose-free milk, or buy Lactaid and add it to your milk and other lactose-containing foods. Lactaid breaks down lactose so that you may be able to eat dairy foods without problems.

People with lactose intolerance who avoid dairy products need to take a calcium supplement. Talk to your health-care provider about the best one for you. Eat vegetables and fruits that contain calcium as well.

There's also a wide variety of yogurts on the market, from full-fat to fat-free regular and Greek yogurt. Choose the lowest-fat types. Be sure to also think about how a yogurt is sweetened. You can find plain regular or Greek yogurt that contains no added sweeteners, as well as fruit-flavored yogurt sweetened with a no-calorie sweetener or with regular sweeteners. Once fruit is added to yogurt, the calories and carbohydrates go up. The calories go up less if the yogurt is sweetened with a no-calorie sweetener. This is also true for yogurt drinks. Skip the sprinkles, granola, and other calorie-raising, low-nutrient additions.

Calcium on the Nutrition Facts Label

According to the Food and Drug Administration's regulations, food labels must provide daily values for calcium. As a result, the calcium content of many foods you buy is easy to figure out because the daily value for calcium is 1,000 mg per day. For example, if a product contains 35% of the daily value of calcium per serving, you know that the serving provides 350 mg of calcium. (Learn more about daily values in chapter 7.)

People who have difficulty getting enough calcium may need to take a calcium supplement. This is especially true for women of child-bearing years, postmenopausal women, and people who eat fewer than 1,500 calories a day. If you do not eat enough calcium, talk to your health-care provider about using a calcium supplement and ask for help selecting the best one for you. Choose a capsule, tablet, or bite-size chewable calcium supplement that provides 500 mg. If you need two, take them at different times of the day to maximize absorption, and take them at a time different from a multivitamin, if you take one. The body can't absorb more than 500 mg at a time.

To properly absorb the calcium you get, you also need enough vitamin D. If you drink 3 servings of milk a day and take a daily multivitamin and mineral supplement with 400 IU of vitamin D, you'll get enough vitamin D. Another way to easily get more vitamin D is to buy a calcium supplement that also contains vitamin D.

Tips for Buying, Preparing, and Eating More Milks and Yogurts

- Drink 8 ounces of fat-free fortified milk at meals.
- Gradually switch to fat-free milk to lower your saturated and trans fats and calories.
- Add a bit more milk to coffee or tea if you use it.
- Choose fat-free milk when you order a fancy coffee or tea drink.
- Eat more hot cereal, substitute milk for at least half (if not all) the water you use to cook the cereal, or use more milk on the cereal as you eat it.
- Eat more high-fiber dry cereals. You'll consume more milk and get a good boost of fiber. Choose cereals that are calcium-fortified.
- Don't limit cereal and milk to breakfast; it can be a quick-and-easy lunch, dinner, or snack. It is a great way to work in another fruit serving, too.
- Blend a milkshake or yogurt shake for a quick and tasty breakfast or snack. Put a serving of milk or yogurt in a blender, add a serving of fruit (banana, strawberries, or peaches), add a bit of extract (vanilla, rum, or maple), blend it up, and sip it down. If you want a cold shake, freeze the fruit before blending.
- Create your own yogurt combo. Take fat-free plain yogurt and add a high-fiber cereal, low-fat granola, dried fruit (diced dried apricots, apples, or pears), or a few chopped nuts for crunch.
- Put a few tablespoons of yogurt on fresh or canned fruit.
- Use plain regular or Greek yogurt as a substitute for sour cream on potatoes. Mix in fresh herbs, garlic, Dijon mustard, cayenne, curry, or any combination of herbs and spices for some extra kick.

- Make yogurt cheese the thickness of cream cheese and add some no-sugar jelly to spread on bagels or toast. Greek yogurt may be thick enough for you. (Make yogurt cheese by draining plain yogurt through cheesecloth for a few hours to remove the liquid.)

- Add fat-free dry milk to recipes where the taste will blend in: meatloaf or meatballs, soups, casseroles, or gravies.

- Add fat-free milk or fat-free dry milk to eggs for scrambled eggs, omelets, or French toast.

TABLE 11.1 Serving Sizes, Calories, and Nutrients for Milks and Yogurts

Food	Serving Size
FAT-FREE MILKS/LOW-FAT MILKS	
Acidophilus milk, fat-free	1 cup
Buttermilk, fat-free	1 cup
Buttermilk, low-fat (1%)	1 cup
Lactaid, fat-free	1 cup
Milk, 1% (low-fat)	1 cup
Milk, evaporated, fat-free	1/2 cup
Milk, fat-free (nonfat, skim)	1 cup
Yogurt, fat-free, flavored, sweetened with Splenda	1 container (6 oz)
Yogurt, fat-free plain	1 container (6 oz)
Yogurt, Greek, fat-free	2/3 cup (6 oz)
Yogurt, low-fat plain	1 container (6 oz)
REDUCED-FAT MILKS	
Acidophilus milk, 2%	1 cup
Kefir, made with 2% milk	1 cup
Lactaid, reduced-fat	1 cup
Milk, reduced-fat (2%)	1 cup
WHOLE MILKS	
Milk, evaporated, whole	1/2 cup
Milk, goat, whole	1 cup
Milk, whole	1 cup
Yogurt, plain, made from whole milk	1 cup
DAIRY-LIKE FOODS	
Chocolate milk, fat-free	1 cup
Chocolate milk, whole	1 cup
Eggnog, whole milk	1/2 cup
Rice drink, fat-free or 1%, plain	1 cup
Rice drink, low-fat, flavored	1 cup
Smoothie, regular, yogurt-based, flavored	1 container (10 fl oz)

Calories	Carb (g)	Fat (g)	Protein (g)
90	13.0	0.2	9.0
98	11.7	0.0	8.1
98	11.7	2.2	8.1
80	13.0	0.0	8.1
110	13.0	2.5	8.0
100	14.5	0.3	9.7
90	13.0	0.2	9.0
80	11.0	0.3	7.0
82	12.0	0.3	8.2
90	6.0	0.0	15.0
107	12.0	2.6	8.9
128	11.2	4.7	7.9
120	13.0	4.6	9.0
130	13.0	5.0	7.9
130	12.0	5.0	8.1
169	12.7	9.5	8.6
168	10.9	10.1	8.7
150	12.0	8.0	8.0
160	12.0	8.0	9.0
160	31.0	0.0	9.0
208	25.9	8.5	7.9
171	17.2	9.5	4.8
90	18.0	1.5	1.1
122	25.0	2.0	1.0
260	49.7	3.3	8.0

continued

TABLE 11.1 *continued*

Food	Serving Size
Soy milk, light	1 cup (8 fl oz)
Soy milk, regular, plain	1 cup
Yogurt and juice blend	1 cup
Yogurt, low-carb, sweetened with Splenda	1 container (6 oz)
Yogurt with fruit, low-fat	1 container (6 oz)

Source: Adapted from *Choose Your Foods: Food Lists for Diabetes.* Academy of Nutrition and Dietetics and American Diabetes Association, 2014.

Calories	Carb (g)	Fat (g)	Protein (g)
100	15.0	2.0	5.0
115	11.0	4.1	8.0
150	34.0	0.0	3.0
70	5.0	3.0	5.0
150	28.0	1.5	6.0

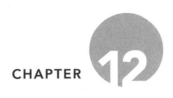

CHAPTER 12

Protein Foods

What's Ahead?

→ Nutrition benefits and drawbacks of protein.

→ Healthy eating goals for the protein group.

→ Assessing how many protein servings you eat now.

→ The ideal number of servings of protein.

→ Tips to help you buy, prepare, and eat healthier sources and smaller amounts of protein.

→ Serving sizes and nutrition numbers for protein.

Foods in the Protein Group

The protein group contains the foods that provide you with most of the animal and plant sources of protein you eat: red meats (beef, lamb, veal, and pork); poultry (chicken and turkey); seafood (shellfish and fish); eggs; cheese; nut spreads, such as peanut and cashew butter (note: nuts are in the fat group, but they contain a good bit of protein, too); plant-based protein foods (legumes such as lentils, refried beans, also found in the starch group due to their carbohydrate content); and soy-based foods (burgers, tempeh, and tofu).

Nutrition Benefits and Drawbacks

This is the first food group discussed in the book for which a key nutrition message is to eat smaller amounts and to show a preference for different types. This is also the first time you'll see a food's nutrition assets followed by its liabilities. The calories from foods in the protein group come from a relatively consistent amount of protein but varied amounts and types of fat. For example, very lean meats, like white fish or turkey breast, provide calories mainly from protein, whereas high-fat protein foods, like full-fat cheese and pork spareribs, provide a similar amount of protein but a good bit of fat, quite possibly unhealthy saturated fat.

Protein foods have plenty of nutrition assets. Your body needs protein. Protein foods provide varying amounts of amino acids (the building blocks of protein) to maintain your bones, muscles, enzymes, and hormones. Red meats, like beef, veal, lamb, and pork, as well as seafood and poultry, are also sources of several vitamins and minerals, such as iron, zinc, thiamine, riboflavin, niacin, magnesium, phosphorus, and vitamins E, B_6, and B_{12}. Cheese is an excellent source of calcium. Fatty fish, such as salmon, tuna, and mackerel, are good sources of the healthy omega-3 fats. Protein foods also have been shown to take longer to digest and, therefore, may keep you feeling fuller or satiated longer.

The plant-based proteins also have a number of nutrition assets. In addition to protein, foods like beans and lentils offer fiber, potassium, and disease-fighting phytonutrients with no saturated fat or cholesterol, unless you add it.

The nutrition liabilities of proteins are their total fat and calorie content as well as their saturated fat and cholesterol content, both of which can raise your LDL (bad) cholesterol and blood lipid levels.

Full-fat cheese (regular, not reduced- or low-fat) and beef contribute the most saturated fat to the average person's diet. Poultry contributes some, but it's way down the list. Eating less cheese and red meat, or choosing lower-fat varieties, is a good first step to help you lower your saturated fat intake. Cholesterol is only found in foods of animal origin, so it stands to reason that many of the protein foods with an animal origin contain cholesterol. Foods with the highest cholesterol content are whole eggs (it's the yolk that contains the cholesterol), organ meats (such as kidney and liver), calamari (squid), and shrimp. All meats, cheese, poultry, and seafood contain some cholesterol. Foods that are high in saturated fat aren't necessarily high in cholesterol. Learn more about all types of fats in chapter 13.

Protein Foods: How Much and What

People generally eat too much protein—nearly double what's thought to be about right for good health. Historically, chowing down on large servings of meat has been a way to show wealth. Our eating habits have evolved to make protein foods the focal point of meals. Along with eating portions of protein foods that are too large, people tend to choose protein foods that are high in total fat and saturated fat, such as full-fat cheese, marbled red meat, sausage, and bacon. The health advice of many nutrition experts today is to eat smaller amounts of protein foods and to choose lean foods to minimize total fat, particularly saturated fat.

A way to eat smaller portions of protein foods is to follow the lead of other cultures. Consider the Chinese stir-fry, in which bite-size tidbits of protein foods are scattered among a greater amount of vegetables and served on top of rice, or Mexican chili, in which a tomato-and-bean base has bits of beef, pork, or sausage in it. Do keep in mind that Americans have Americanized some of these dishes and in turn made them more protein packed and less vegetable dense.

One more tip. Eat more plant-based sources of protein.

Get to Know Yourself

If you want to change your eating habits, you need to assess your current eating habits. Ask yourself these questions about the protein foods you eat:

- How many times a day do I eat protein?
- Do I believe I need to eat protein at every meal for adequate nutrition or blood glucose control?
- Do I ever eat plant-based protein or enjoy a meatless meal?
- What cuts of red meats do I buy? Are they high in fat or lean?
- Do I pull the skin off poultry?
- Do I consume enough seafood, particularly fish high in omega-3 fats?
- What cooking methods, sauces, and seasonings do I use to prepare protein foods?
- What are my typical protein portion sizes at breakfast, lunch, dinner, and snack time at home and at restaurants?

How Many Proteins Servings for You?

In chapter 6, you determined which calorie range was the best for you to follow. Find that calorie range in Table 6.1, and then spot the ounces of protein to eat each day. It should be somewhere between 5 and 9 ounces. Yes, you may easily be able to eat this amount in one sitting, but this is enough protein for an entire day.

Get to Know Your Serving Sizes

Table 12.1 at the end of the chapter (starting on page 162) shows the calories, protein, total fat, saturated fat, and cholesterol per serving for many common proteins. One serving of protein food has about 7 grams of protein, no matter what type of protein food it is. Animal sources of protein do not contain any carbohydrate (unless it's added in preparation). Plant-based sources of proteins like tofu, beans, or peas do contain carbohydrates. The amount of carbohydrate in these foods varies, as you'll see in Table 12.1. Also, don't forget to check out the Nutrition Facts labels on products.

In general, a protein serving is:

- 1 ounce of meat, fish, or cheese.
- 1 egg.
- 1/3–1/2 cup of beans (contains carbohydrate).
- 4 ounces of tofu (contains carbohydrate).

To eat the number of calories you shoot for each day, it's important to eat the correct serving sizes. To do so, weigh and measure your foods at least occasionally to make sure you are estimating correctly.

Sample Meal Plan

The sample meal plan below gives you an idea of how to fit 6 protein servings into an eating plan with 1,400–1,600 calories a day. You'll see that the servings of protein are in bold for quick identification. Chapter 6 provides sample plans and nutrition information for the other calorie ranges.

ONE-DAY MEAL PLAN: **1,400–1,600 CALORIES**

BREAKFAST

1 whole-grain bagel thin (2 oz) with	2 starch
1 1/2 Tbsp light cream cheese	1 fat
3/4 cup blueberries with	1 fruit
1/3 cup fat-free plain yogurt	1/2 milk

LUNCH

Tuna salad made with

3 oz tuna (1/2 cup), water-packed	**3 ounces protein**
1 Tbsp light mayonnaise	1 fat
2 Tbsp diced celery	1 vegetable
1 Tbsp diced onions	
Tomato slices and lettuce leaves	1 free food
1 whole-wheat tortilla	2 starch
1 cup baby carrots	1 vegetable
1 cup fat-free milk	1 milk

DINNER

3 oz grilled salmon with	**3 ounces protein**
lemon and herbs	free food
Stir-fried vegetables with	
1/4 cup onions, cooked	2 vegetable
1/2 cup snow peas, cooked	
1/2 cup red peppers, cooked	
2 tsp canola oil	2 fats
2/3 cup brown rice	3 starch

EVENING SNACK

Mix together:

1/2 cup crushed canned pineapple (packed in own juice)	1 fruit
1/3 cup fat-free plain yogurt	1/2 milk
1/8 cup chopped pecans	2 fat

Protein and Diabetes

Learn more about the types of foods with protein and fat recommended for people with diabetes in chapter 3. The biggest reason to eat smaller portions of protein and to change the types of protein you select is to cut down on your intake of total fat, saturated fat, and cholesterol. Diabetes increases your risk of heart disease and high blood pressure. Reducing your saturated fat and cholesterol intake can help improve your blood lipid levels.

Fat and Calories in Protein Foods

The amount of fat in foods is what creates the big calorie differences between different protein foods. Protein foods fit into four subgroups: lean, medium-fat, high-fat, and plant-based. See Table 12.2 for examples of each.

Choose Lean

Red Meats. Choose lean options for all types of red meat. Select-grade meats are leanest, choice cuts contain moderate fat, and prime cuts contain the most fat. Regardless of grade, look for well-trimmed cuts or trim them well before you cook them. Table 12.3 gives some leaner options.

Poultry. Chicken and turkey are lower in fat than most red meats and contain less saturated fat, particularly when you remove the

TABLE 12.2	Types and Examples of Protein Foods		
Type of Protein	Fat (g)*	Calories*	Examples
Lean	0–2	25–45	Poultry (without skin), beef (tenderloin, sirloin, or ground round, 90% or higher lean/10% or lower fat), or seafood (salmon, tuna, tilapia, or shellfish)
Medium-fat	3–7	55–75	Beef trimmed of visible fat: ground beef (85% or higher lean/15% or lower fat), prime cuts of beef, pork cutlet, egg, cheese (string, feta, part-skim, reduced-fat)
High-fat	8+	100	Pork spareribs, bacon, and regular cheese
Plant-based	Varies+	Varies+	Legumes, tofu, nut spreads

*Nutrition information is per 1 ounce cooked or 1 serving for portions not measured in ounces, like legumes. Plant-based protein foods often contains some carbohydrate.

Source: Adapted from Choose Your Foods: Food Lists for Diabetes. Academy of Nutrition and Dietetics and American Diabetes Association, 2014.

TABLE 12.3	Leaner and Higher-Fat Cuts of Red Meat	
Type of Red Meat	Leaner Cuts	Higher-Fat Cuts
Beef	Round steaks and roasts (round eye, top round, bottom round, round tip), top loin, top sirloin, chuck shoulder and arm roasts, flank steak, skirt steak, top loin, ground beef (90% lean or greater)	Rib eye steak, rib roast, short ribs, ground beef (less than 90% lean)
Lamb	Leg, loin chop	Ground lamb, blade
Pork	Loin, tenderloin, center loin, butterfly-cut chops, loin rib chops, ham	Spareribs, country ribs, sausage, bacon
Veal	Varies	Breast

skin. Purchase chicken or turkey without skin or remove the skin before you cook it. White-meat chicken (the breast) is lower in fat than dark meat (thigh and leg) by a small margin; however, if you enjoy dark meat more, the difference isn't that great. Just eat less of it. If you purchase cooked chicken and turkey, remove the skin and as much fat as possible before you eat it. More turkey products are available today, including turkey cutlets and breast, ground turkey, and turkey sausage. These are most often lower in fat than their red-meat cousins. When possible, use them to replace red meat or to replace some of the red meat. For example, if you make a meatloaf, consider using half lean ground beef and half ground turkey. Duck and Cornish hen are higher in fat than chicken and turkey.

Seafood. Most shellfish and fish are lower in fat and saturated fat than red meat; however, their fat content varies. Some of the white fishes (flounder, sole, and haddock) are very lean, whereas salmon, mackerel, and bluefish have more fat. Some of the fat in these fattier fish is the healthier omega-3 fat. Buy tuna packed in water rather than tuna packed in oil, and enjoy canned salmon as a healthy alternative to tuna.

Also avoid premade salads like tuna fish, seafood, and egg salad. These tend to be loaded with mayonnaise, which adds unwanted calories.

Luncheon, Cold Cuts, and Breakfast Meats. Eat fewer processed meats and poultry products to lighten your sodium count and cut down on ingredients like preservatives. If you need to follow a low-sodium eating plan, you may want to avoid these foods altogether. At least try to buy low-sodium varieties of these foods if they're available. When you do purchase these foods, consider these tips.

- Choose the lowest in fat.

- Choose turkey, smoked turkey, turkey ham, roast beef, or ham.

- Avoid high-fat luncheon meats like salami, bologna, and capacola.

- Choose lean hot dogs or those made from turkey.

- With breakfast meats, such as sausage or bacon, choose leaner and lower-fat options.

Cheese. Full-fat cheese tops the list of foods high in saturated fat. If you're a big cheese eater—say, a couple of ounces a day—save calories and grams of fat and saturated fat by making healthier selections, like reduced-fat, part-skim, or low-fat versions, but do make sure you enjoy the taste. It's easy to find lower-fat versions of many hard and soft cheeses, such as mozzarella, Jarlsberg, ricotta, and cottage cheese.

Plant-based. Beans, peas, and lentils are cost-effective sources of protein that come in many varieties. They are excellent sources of fiber and are low in fat and contain no cholesterol. Buy them dried, canned, frozen, or fresh. Canned varieties can be high in sodium, so look for reduced-sodium options and drain and rinse them to remove even more sodium. Nut spreads, such as almond butter and peanut butter, are high in fat but contain no cholesterol and minimal saturated fat (a serving of 1 tablespoon or more can be considered a protein serving; if less than that, it should be considered a serving of fat). Plus, a little goes a long way. Tofu is another good protein option that can be added to soups, stir-fries, and even smoothies.

Prepare Low Fat

How you prepare your protein foods is a critical step to keeping them low in fat and calories. Trim off any visible fat from red meats. Use cooking techniques that use no or only a small amount of oil, butter, mayonnaise, or cream. Learn to use low- or no-calorie sauces, flavorings, and seasonings. Use a cooking method that drips and drains fat rather than adds it, such as barbecuing, grilling, or poaching.

Here are some tips to reduce fat during food preparation.

- Grill with different flavored wood chips, such as mesquite or hickory.

- Poach in broth, wine, or sherry. Add garlic, herbs, or any combination of flavors to the poaching liquid.

- Marinate meat, chicken, or fish for at least several hours in fat-free ingredients before cooking. Try sherry, mustard, and garlic; soy or teriyaki sauce (note: these are high in sodium); ginger and garlic; vinegar (any variety); or garlic and basil.

- Make low-fat gravy using the drippings from baking or roasting as follows: Refrigerate the drippings until the fat turns solid and floats to the top. Remove the fat with a spoon. Then put the drippings in a pan, add a bit of flour or cornstarch with a whisk, and heat to thicken. You can also purée any celery, onion, or carrots that were in the roasting pan and add them to the defatted gravy mixture to thicken. You may want to purchase a fat separator, which is a strainer that allows you to pour the juices out and leave the fat in the container. One of these can really help you save time.

- Use salsa or pico de gallo to spice up ground beef, chicken, or shrimp for fajitas, burritos, or soft tacos.

- Mix fat-free plain yogurt with mustard and dill to top fish.

- Make low-fat tartar sauce with low-fat or fat-free mayonnaise and relish.

Eat Less

Downsize Your Portions. If your usual animal protein portion has typically been more than 4, 6, or 8 ounces at a meal, then 3 ounces may seem tiny at first. To have long-term success, downsize slowly, 1 ounce at a time. If you usually eat 5 or 6 ounces of turkey in a sandwich, step down to 4 ounces and then down to 3 ounces over the course of a few months. This is harder to do in protein-focused restaurant meals, but the techniques of splitting and sharing can help. Stuff sandwiches with lettuce, tomato, sliced cucumber, and sprouts to bulk them up and eat more vegetables. When you downsize servings, weigh items more frequently to help your eyes adjust. Even if your servings are a bit larger than desirable in the beginning, choosing lean cuts and preparing food in low-fat ways are moves in a healthy, calorie-reducing direction.

Weigh and Measure. It is important to weigh protein foods. Use a food scale as often as possible to make sure your portions are the right size and don't slowly get larger. It is easy to cut a slightly bigger wedge of cheese or put an extra ounce of meat in a sandwich. The more often you weigh your portions of meat before they go in your mouth, the more often you'll eat the correct portion. Plus, you'll be a better guesstimater at restaurants.

Another way to estimate protein portions is to think in terms of common objects. The palm of your hand—both width and depth—is about the size of a 3-ounce piece of meat. You can also think of a standard deck of playing cards or computer mouse to visually estimate 3 ounces of cooked meat.

Measuring from Raw to Cooked

Here are quick rules to translate from raw to cooked servings:

- Raw meat with no bone: 4 ounces raw = 3 ounces cooked.

- Raw meat with bone: 5 ounces raw = 3 ounces cooked.

- Raw poultry with bone and skin: 4 1/4 to 4 1/2 ounces raw = 3 ounces cooked. The skin accounts for 1/4 to 1/2 ounce. (Remove skin before cooking or before serving to reduce the fat, saturated fat, and cholesterol content.)

When you order meats in restaurants, observe that they refer to the raw weight. For example a quarter-pound hamburger equals 3 ounces cooked; a 10-ounce T-bone steak equals about 6 ounces cooked.

Here's another helpful tip. Think about the portions you want to eat when you purchase foods in the supermarket. For example, if you buy lean turkey for sandwiches and you want to make four sandwiches, each with 3 ounces of turkey, then buy 12 ounces. If you buy too much, then you are likely to overeat. Apply this same logic to all the meats, poultry, and seafood you buy and control your portions before you even put the food on the table. Portion control is further covered in chapter 20.

Easy Ways to Eat Less

- Split sandwiches in restaurants. Ask for two extra pieces of bread or an extra roll, and split the meat from one sandwich into two.

- Split a meat entrée in restaurants. The usual portion you are served in sit-down restaurants is 6–8 ounces or more. This is plenty for two. If you need more food, fill the meal out with an extra salad, cooked vegetable, or healthy starch.

- Make room on your plate for starches and vegetables, so that the smaller-than-usual piece of meat won't seem so small.

- Buy and prepare smaller quantities (just what you need for the recipe) so you eat less.

- Cook dishes that stretch the meat portion: Chinese stir-fry, pasta with meat sauce, or beef and bean burritos.

- Load sandwiches with raw vegetables. (Using pita bread makes this easy because you can stuff the pocket.)

- In fast-food restaurants, order single-, regular-, or junior-size sandwiches and stay away from the doubles and triples.

- Start the day with a meatless breakfast.

- Join the "meatless Monday" movement and designate one day a week, perhaps Mondays, as a meatless day, during which you'll enjoy only plant-based sources of protein.

TABLE 12.1 Protein Serving Sizes, Calories, and Nutrients	
Food	Serving Size
LEAN PROTEIN	
Beef jerky, dried	0.5 oz
Beef tenderloin, lean, broiled	1 oz
Beef, chipped, dried	1 oz
Beef, chuck, pot roast, lean only, cooked	1 oz
Beef, cubed steak, lean, cooked	1 oz
Beef, flank steak, lean, cooked	1 oz
Beef, ground round, cooked	1 oz
Beef, rib roast, lean, roasted	1 oz
Beef, round steak, lean, cooked	1 oz
Beef, rump roast, cooked	1 oz
Beef, sirloin, lean, cooked	1 oz
Beef, top round, braised	1 oz
Buffalo (bison), roasted	1 oz
Canadian bacon, grilled	1 oz
Catfish fillet, cooked	1 oz
Cheese, American, fat-free	1 slice
Cheese, American, reduced-fat	1 oz
Cheese, cheddar, fat-free	1 oz
Cheese, feta, fat-free, plain	1 oz
Cheese, mozzarella, fat-free	1 oz
Cheese, ricotta, fat-free	1/4 cup
Cheese, Swiss, fat-free	1 oz
Chicken breast, meat only, cooked	1 oz
Chicken, dark meat, no skin, roasted	1 oz
Clams, fresh, cooked	1 oz
Cod fillet, cooked	1 oz
Cornish game hen, cooked, no skin	1 oz
Cottage cheese, creamed, 4.5% milkfat	1/4 cup
Cottage cheese, fat-free	1/4 cup

Calories	Protein (g)	Fat (g)	Saturated Fat (g)	Cholesterol (mg)
58	4.7	3.6	1.5	7
55	8.1	2.2	0.8	22
47	8.2	1.1	0.0	12
61	9.3	2.3	0.9	29
57	8.9	2.2	0.7	27
53	7.9	2.1	0.9	14
57	10.3	1.4	0.5	26
65	7.7	3.5	1.4	23
61	9.6	2.2	0.8	29
59	8.9	2.3	0.8	27
52	8.6	1.6	0.6	16
56	10.2	1.4	0.5	26
41	8.1	0.7	0.3	23
52	6.9	2.4	0.8	16
43	5.3	2.3	0.5	18
30	5.0	0.0	0.0	3
68	5.4	4.0	2.5	14
45	9.0	0.0	0.0	3
30	6.0	0.0	0.0	0
45	7.9	0.0	0.0	4
45	8.0	0.0	0.0	20
41	6.8	0.0	0.0	7
47	8.8	1.0	0.3	24
58	7.7	2.8	0.8	26
42	7.2	0.6	0.1	19
30	6.5	0.2	0.0	16
38	6.6	1.1	0.3	30
54	6.5	2.3	1.0	8
40	7.0	0.0	0.0	3

continued

TABLE 12.1 *continued*

Food	Serving Size
Cottage cheese, low-fat, 1% milkfat	1/4 cup
Crab, steamed	1 oz
Duck, domestic, no skin, roasted	1 oz
Egg substitute (Egg Beaters)	1/4 cup
Egg whites	2 egg whites
Flounder, cooked	1 oz
Goose, no skin, roasted	1 oz
Haddock, cooked	1 oz
Halibut fillet, cooked	1 oz
Ham, boiled, lean, deli–sandwich type (≤3 g fat/oz)	1 oz
Ham, canned, fully cooked	1 oz
Ham, cured, roasted	1 oz
Ham, extra lean (95% fat-free)	1 oz
Heart, beef, cooked	1 oz
Herring, smoked	1 oz
Hot dog or frankfurter (≤3 g fat/oz)	1 frankfurter
Kidney, beef, cooked	1 oz
Lamb leg, sirloin, roast, lean	1 oz
Lamb loin, roast or chop, cooked	1 oz
Liver, chicken, cooked	1 oz
Lobster, fresh, steamed	1 oz
Lox (smoked salmon)	1 oz
Orange roughy, cooked, dry heat	1 oz
Ostrich, cooked	1 oz
Oysters, cooked	6 medium
Pork chop, cooked	1 oz
Pork tenderloin, cooked	1 oz
Rabbit, cooked	1 oz
Salmon, canned, solids and liquids	1 oz
Salmon, fresh, broiled or baked	1 oz

Calories	Protein (g)	Fat (g)	Saturated Fat (g)	Cholesterol (mg)
41	7.0	0.6	0.4	2
29	5.7	0.5	0.1	28
57	6.6	3.2	1.0	25
30	6.0	0.0	0.0	0
33	6.9	0.0	0.0	0
33	6.8	0.4	0.1	19
67	8.2	3.6	1.0	27
32	6.9	0.3	0.0	21
40	7.6	0.8	0.1	12
29	4.5	1.0	0.5	15
64	5.8	4.3	1.4	18
44	7.1	1.6	0.5	16
30	4.5	1.0	0.4	14
50	8.1	1.6	0.0	55
61	7.0	3.5	1.0	23
70	6.0	2.5	1.0	20
45	7.7	1.3	0.3	203
58	8.0	2.6	0.9	26
61	8.5	2.8	1.0	27
47	6.9	1.8	0.6	159
28	5.8	0.2	0.0	20
33	5.2	1.2	0.3	6
30	6.4	0.3	0.0	23
40	7.6	0.8	0.0	27
46	4.1	1.2	0.4	22
57	8.4	2.4	0.9	24
40	7.4	1.0	0.3	21
58	8.6	2.4	0.7	24
39	5.6	1.7	0.4	16
61	7.7	3.1	0.5	25

continued

TABLE 12.1 *continued*

Food	Serving Size
Sardines, packed in oil, drained	2 small (2 2/3" x 1/2" x 1/4")
Sausage, smoked (≤3 g fat/oz)	1 oz
Scallops, fresh, steamed	1 oz
Shellfish, imitation	1 oz
Shrimp, fresh, cooked in water	1 oz
Steak, porterhouse, lean, broiled	1 oz
Steak, T-bone, lean, broiled	1 oz
Tilapia fillet, cooked	1 oz
Trout, cooked	1 oz
Tuna, canned in oil, drained	1 oz
Tuna, canned in water, drained	1 oz
Tuna, fresh, cooked	1 oz
Turkey breast (cutlet), no skin, roasted	1 oz
Turkey ham (≤3 g fat/oz)	1 oz
Turkey kielbasa (≤3 g fat/oz)	1 oz
Turkey pastrami (≤3 g fat/oz)	1 oz
Turkey, dark meat, no skin, cooked	1 oz
Veal loin, chop, cooked	1 oz
Veal roast	1 oz
Venison (deer), roast	1 oz
MEDIUM-FAT PROTEIN	
Beef patty, ground, extra lean, pan broiled (85% lean)	1 oz
Beef patty, ground, lean, pan broiled (80% lean)	1 oz
Beef patty, ground, regular, pan broiled (75% lean)	1 oz
Beef, prime rib, roasted	1 oz
Beef, short ribs, cooked	1 oz
Cheese spread	1 oz
Cheese, Colby Jack, reduced-fat	1 oz
Cheese, feta, regular	1 oz

Calories	Protein (g)	Fat (g)	Saturated Fat (g)	Cholesterol (mg)
50	5.9	2.7	0.4	34
40	3.5	1.3	0.5	12
32	6.6	0.4	0.0	15
29	3.4	0.4	0.0	6
28	5.9	0.3	0.1	55
60	7.5	3.1	1.1	19
57	7.6	2.8	1.0	16
37	7.4	0.8	0.3	25
54	7.5	2.4	0.4	21
53	7.5	2.3	0.0	9
33	7.2	0.2	0.1	8
52	8.5	1.8	0.5	14
38	8.5	0.2	0.1	23
36	5.4	1.4	0.0	16
45	4.0	2.5	1.0	16
40	5.2	1.8	1.0	15
53	8.1	2.0	1.0	24
64	9.5	2.6	0.7	35
55	9.0	1.9	0.5	33
45	8.5	0.9	0.4	32
66	7.0	4.0	1.6	24
68	6.8	4.5	1.7	24
70	6.6	4.7	1.8	23
83	7.7	5.5	2.4	23
84	8.7	5.1	2.2	26
82	4.6	6.0	3.8	16
80	7.0	5.0	3.5	15
75	4.0	6.0	4.2	25

continued

TABLE 12.1 *continued*

Food	Serving Size
Cheese, Mexican, reduced-fat	1 oz
Cheese, Monterey Jack, reduced-fat	1 oz
Cheese, mozzarella (part skim milk)	1 oz
Cheese, mozzarella, reduced-fat	1 oz
Cheese, ricotta (part skim milk)	1/4 cup
Cheese, string	1 oz
Cheese, Swiss, reduced-fat	1 oz
Chicken, with skin, roasted	1 oz
Chicken, meat and skin, fried, flour coated	1 oz
Corned beef brisket, cooked	1 oz
Dove, cooked	1 oz
Duck, wild, meat and skin (not cooked)	1 oz
Egg, fresh	1 egg
Fish, fried, cornmeal coating	1 oz
Goose, wild, with skin, cooked	1 oz
Lamb rib, roasted	1 oz
Lamb, ground, broiled	1 oz
Meatloaf	1 oz
Pheasant (grouse), cooked, meat and skin	1 oz
Pork cutlet, cooked	1 oz
Pork, Boston blade, roasted	1 oz
Sausage, hard (<5 g fat/oz)	1 oz
Tongue (beef), cooked	1 oz
Turkey, ground, cooked	1 oz
Veal cutlet, lean, cooked	1 oz
HIGH-FAT PROTEIN	
Bacon, fried, drained	2 slices (16 per lb)
Bacon, turkey	3 slices
Bologna	1 oz
Cheese, American	1 oz

Calories	Protein (g)	Fat (g)	Saturated Fat (g)	Cholesterol (mg)
81	8.1	6.0	3.0	20
80	7.0	6.0	3.5	20
72	6.9	4.5	2.9	18
70	8.0	4.0	2.5	15
85	7.0	4.9	3.0	19
83	7.1	5.3	3.5	18
70	9.0	3.5	2.0	10
68	7.7	3.8	1.1	25
76	8.1	4.2	1.1	25
71	5.1	5.4	1.8	28
62	6.8	3.7	1.1	33
60	4.9	4.3	1.4	23
74	6.3	5.0	1.5	212
65	5.1	3.8	1.0	23
86	7.1	6.2	1.9	26
66	7.4	3.8	1.3	25
80	7.0	5.6	2.3	27
65	6.0	3.9	1.5	17
70	9.2	3.4	1.0	25
71	7.9	4.2	1.5	24
76	6.5	5.3	2.0	24
45	4.0	2.5	1.0	15
80	5.5	6.3	2.3	37
67	7.7	3.7	1.0	29
57	10.4	1.4	0.5	38
85	5.9	6.6	2.2	17
92	7.1	6.7	2.0	24
90	3.3	8.0	3.0	16
106	6.3	8.9	5.6	27

continued

TABLE 12.1 *continued*

Food	Serving Size
Cheese, blue-veined (blue, Roquefort)	1 oz
Cheese, cheddar-type	1 oz
Cheese, goat, hard	1 oz
Cheese, Monterey Jack	1 oz
Cheese, Parmesan	1 oz
Cheese, Swiss, regular	1 oz
Chorizo sausage, cooked	1 oz
Hot dog (wiener, frankfurter)	1 hot dog (10/lb)
Hot dog, chicken	1 hot dog (10/lb)
Hot dog, turkey	1 hot dog (10/lb)
Pastrami, regular	1 oz
Pork sausage, cooked	1 oz
Pork spareribs, cooked, lean and fat	1 oz
Pork, ground, cooked	1 oz
Queso asadero (Mexican melting cheese)	1 oz
Salami, hard	1 oz
Sausage, bratwurst, fresh, cooked	1 oz
Sausage, Italian, cooked	1 oz
Sausage, knockwurst, cooked	1 oz
Sausage, Polish	1 oz
Sausage, smoked	1 oz
Sausage, summer	1 oz
PLANT-BASED PROTEINS (For Beans, Peas, and Lentils See Starch List)	
Almond butter, plain	1 Tbsp
"Bacon" strips, soy-based	3 strips
Breakfast patty, meatless (soy-based)	1 patty (1 1/2 oz)
Cashew butter, plain	1 Tbsp
"Chicken" nuggets, breaded (soy-based)	2 nuggets (1 1/2 oz)
Edamame	1/2 cup

Calories	Protein (g)	Fat (g)	Saturated Fat (g)	Cholesterol (mg)
100	6.1	8.2	5.0	21
114	7.1	9.4	6.0	30
127	8.6	10.0	6.9	30
106	7.0	8.6	5.0	25
110	10.0	7.0	4.0	20
108	7.6	7.9	5.0	26
95	3.5	8.5	3.0	20
137	5.2	12.4	4.8	22
116	5.8	8.8	2.5	45
102	6.4	8.0	2.7	48
99	4.9	8.3	3.0	26
104	5.6	8.8	3.1	23
112	8.2	8.6	3.2	34
84	7.3	5.9	2.2	27
101	6.4	8.0	5.1	30
105	7.4	8.2	3.1	28
97	4.7	7.4	2.7	19
91	5.7	7.3	3.0	22
87	3.4	7.9	3.0	16
92	4.0	8.1	3.0	20
91	3.4	8.1	2.8	16
95	4.5	8.4	3.0	21
91	2.9	8.6	0.8	0
68	9.0	3.0	0.0	0
79	9.9	2.8	0.5	0
86	2.6	7.2	1.2	0
90	7.0	3.5	0.5	0
95	8.4	4.0	0.5	0

continued

TABLE 12.1 *continued*

Food	Serving Size
Falafel (spiced chickpea and wheat)	3 patties (approx 2 1/4")
Frankfurter (hot dog), meatless (soy-based)	1 frankfurter (1 1/2 oz)
Hummus	1/3 cup
Meatless burger (soy-based)	1 patty (3 oz)
Meatless burger (vegetable and starch–based)	1 patty
Meatless "beef" crumbles (soy-based)	2 oz
Meatless deli slices	1 oz
Meatless "sausage" crumbles (soy-based)	2 oz
Mycoprotein (chicken: tenders or crumbles), meatless	2 oz
Peanut butter, smooth or crunchy	1 Tbsp
Soy nut butter	1 Tbsp
Soy nuts, dry-roasted, no salt	3/4 oz
Tempeh (bean cake)	1/4 cup
Tofu, firm	4 oz (1/2 cup)
Tofu, lite, firm, silken	4 oz (1/2 cup)

Source: Adapted from *Choose Your Foods: Food Lists for Diabetes.* Academy of Nutrition and Dietetics and American Diabetes Association, 2014.

Calories	Protein (g)	Fat (g)	Saturated Fat (g)	Cholesterol (mg)
170	6.8	9.1	1.2	0
70	8.0	2.0	0.0	0
137	6.5	7.9	1.2	0
117	12.0	5.0	0.6	0
130	13.0	3.0	1.0	15
60	13.0	0.5	0.1	0
55	7.0	1.5	0.1	0
60	7.0	0.0	0.0	0
60	7.0	1.0	0.3	0
96	4.0	8.4	1.6	0
96	4.4	8.0	1.0	0
96	8.4	4.6	0.7	0
84	8.0	3.2	0.0	0
80	9.3	4.7	1.0	0
45	7.5	1.5	0.2	0

CHAPTER 13

Fats and Oils

What's Ahead?

- The nutrition benefits and drawbacks of fats and oils.
- Healthy eating goals for fats and oils.
- Assess the servings of fat you eat.
- The ideal number of fat servings for you.
- The different types of fats, how they affect your blood lipids (fats), and how to eat the right amounts.
- Tips to help you choose and use healthier fats and oils.
- Tips for slimming down your favorite recipes.
- Serving sizes and nutrition numbers for fats.

Foods in the Fats and Oils Group

This group includes the fats and oils you use when you prepare or eat foods. It also includes a few foods that contain most of their calories as fat. Some are healthier, like nuts, peanut butter, avocado, and seeds, and some are not so healthy, like bacon and sausage. This group doesn't include the fat that is part of meats, cheese, and other protein foods which contain varying amounts and types of fats. That fat is factored into your food choices from the protein group.

Nutrition Benefits and Drawbacks

While fat has a bad reputation, some types of fats are essential for a healthy body. You need two essential fats, more precisely the fatty acids linoleic acid and alpha-linolenic acid. They're called essential because your body can't make them from other fats you eat. These fatty acids are widely available in foods, and most people have no problem getting enough of them.

One asset of fats and oils is that they are carriers for the fat-soluble vitamins A, D, E, and K and for the category of vitamins called carotenoids, which are essential to health. Fats are also important to maintain healthy skin. Some fatty acids are part of several hormones. Fat provides a source of energy when your primary source of energy, carbohydrate, runs out. Foods that specifically contain omega-3 fats, like certain types of fish, are recommended for everyone, including individuals with diabetes, because they have been shown to reduce the risk of heart disease.

But fat also has its drawbacks. First, it's packed with calories: each gram of fat contains 9 calories. This is more than twice as many as the 4 calories per gram for carbohydrate and protein. As fat is a source of excess calories, eating too much of it can contribute to weight gain. Eating too much saturated fat can also raise your LDL cholesterol and contribute to heart disease, stroke, and insulin resistance.

Fat: Added or Attached?

To see how fat grams can creep into your meals, think of the fats you eat in two categories: "added fats" and "attached fats." Added fats are fats that you use to prepare and eat food—the oil to fry an egg, the mayonnaise in tuna salad, salad dressing on salad, and cream cheese on bagels. Find ways to cut down on these fats and oils. Table 13.1 has some examples to show the difference that adding fats makes.

In foods with attached fats, the fat is simply part of the food and cannot be taken out. For example, there is no way to take the fat out of nuts, peanut butter, eggs, cheese, or avocado. To reduce the amount of fat from these foods, eat less of them or avoid them.

Fats: How Much and What Types People Eat

Americans eat about 35% of their calories as fat. That's on the high end of the recommended range of 20 to 35%, but not extremely high. Do keep in mind that many Americans eat more total calories than they need. Our bigger problem is the type of fat we eat—too much saturated fat, which is no surprise given the amount of red meat, full-fat milk and cheese, ice cream, desserts, and fried restaurant foods we eat. Too much saturated fat can lead to high LDL (bad cholesterol) and an increased risk of heart and blood vessel problems. Trans fats are also a source of saturated fat.

TABLE 13.1 **Nutritional Value of Foods with and without Added Fat**

Food	Serving	Calories	Fat (g)	Sat. Fat (g)	Chol. (mg)
Bread	1 slice	65	1	0	0
Bread *with 1 tsp butter*	1 slice	100	5	2	10
Bread *with 1 tsp margarine*	1 slice	100	5	1	0
Macaroni	1 cup	197	1	0	0
Macaroni *and cheese*	1 cup	430	22	9	42
Chicken breast, roasted, no skin	3 oz	142	3	1	72
Chicken breast, roasted, *with skin*	3 oz	165	7	2	71
Chicken breast, *fried, with skin*	3 oz	218	11	3	71

Get to Know Yourself

If you want to change your eating habits, you need to take stock of your current eating habits. Ask yourself these questions about the fats and oils you eat:

- Which fats and oils do I buy and use?

- Can I buy and use healthier oils and cut down on unhealthy fats and oils?

- How much fat and oil do I use each day in food preparation?

- How much fat and oil do I put on or add to foods at home and in restaurants?

- How often do I eat fried foods?

- What low-fat and fat-free foods do I buy to limit the amount of fat I eat?

- When I eat in restaurants, do I minimize the amount of fat I eat by ordering lower-fat items and limiting added fats?

How Many Fat Servings for You?

In chapter 6, you determined which calorie range was best for you to follow at the moment. Find that calorie range in Table 6.1 and spot the number of fat servings to eat each day. It is somewhere between 5 and 12.

Each fat serving has about 5 grams of fat and 45 calories. Table 13.2 at the end of the chapter (starting on page 190) shows the serving sizes for added fats, along with information on their calories, total fat, type of fats, and cholesterol content.

Because the calories from fat add up very quickly, it is particularly important to pay attention to serving sizes. An extra teaspoon of regular margarine or butter adds 35 calories, and an extra tablespoon of creamy dressing can be an extra 70 or more calories.

Sample Meal Plan

The sample meal plan below gives you an idea of how to fit six servings of fat into your day. The sample is designed for a person who needs 1,400–1,600 calories a day. You'll see that the servings of fats and oils are in bold for quick identification. Chapter 6 provides sample plans for other calorie ranges, along with nutritional information for several plans.

ONE-DAY MEAL PLAN: 1,400–1,600 CALORIES

BREAKFAST

1 whole-grain bagel thin (2 oz) with	2 starch
1 1/2 Tbsp light cream cheese	**1 fat**
3/4 cup blueberries with	1 fruit
1/3 cup fat-free plain yogurt	1/2 milk

LUNCH

Tuna salad made with	
3 oz tuna (1/2 cup), water-packed	3 oz protein
1 Tbsp light mayonnaise	**1 fat**
2 Tbsp diced celery	1 vegetable
1 Tbsp diced onions	
Tomato slices and lettuce leaves	1 free food
1 whole-wheat tortilla	2 starch
1 cup baby carrots	1 vegetable
1 cup fat-free milk	1 milk

DINNER

3 oz grilled salmon with	3 oz protein
lemon and herbs	free food
Stir-fried vegetables with	
1/4 cup onions, cooked	2 vegetable
1/2 cup snow peas, cooked	
1/2 cup red peppers, cooked	
2 tsp canola oil	**2 fat**
2/3 cup brown rice	2 starch

EVENING SNACK
Mix together:

1/2 cup crushed canned pineapple (packed in own juice)	1 fruit
1/3 cup fat-free plain yogurt	1/2 milk
1/8 cup chopped pecans	**2 fat**

Fats and Diabetes

Diabetes increases the risk for high blood pressure and abnormal blood lipids (Table 13.3). Your main focus should be on choosing and eating healthy fats to reduce these risks. Your secondary focus should be on eating less total fat, especially if you believe you eat more than 35% of your calories as fat and want to lose weight. Read more about the current American Diabetes Association recommendations for fat intake in chapter 3 and lipid levels in chapter 1.

Healthy Fats

Nutrition experts now advise you to get most of your calories from fat as a combination of polyunsaturated and monounsaturated fats. Table 13.3 shows how these fats positively affect your blood lipids.

TABLE 13.3 How the Fats You Eat Affect the Fats in Your Blood

Is It Healthy?	Type of Fat in Foods	Effect on Blood Lipids
Unhealthy fat	Saturated fat	↑ total cholesterol ↑ LDL cholesterol
	Trans fat	↑ total cholesterol ↑ LDL cholesterol
Healthy fat	Polyunsaturated fat	↓ total cholesterol ↓ LDL cholesterol ↓ HDL cholesterol
	Monounsaturated	↓ total cholesterol ↓ LDL cholesterol ↑ HDL cholesterol

Polyunsaturated Fats

The two main types of polyunsaturated fats are the omega-3 fats and omega-6 fats. Both are good for your heart and blood lipids. Omega-3 polyunsaturated fats have been shown to reduce the overall risk of heart disease by lowering triglycerides and reducing the "stickiness" of blood platelets so that they don't stick to your artery walls. Liquid vegetable oils, such as corn, soybean, and sunflower oils, contain mainly omega-6 polyunsaturated fats. Omega-3 fats are found in both plant and animal fats. The plant sources of

Tips for Eating More Omega-3 and Omega-6 Fats

Get More Omega-3

- Eat fattier fish at least two times a week: salmon, trout, albacore tuna, sardines, eel, herring, and mackerel.

- Sprinkle ground flaxseed on dry or cooked cereal, in casseroles, or on salads. Eat more walnuts or use walnut oil. Enjoy a small handful of walnuts as a snack, or make a homemade salad dressing with walnut oil.

Get More Omega-6

- Choose processed foods (when you eat them) made with healthier oils that aren't partially hydrogenated.

- Use healthier oils in cooking, and use these instead of solid fat whenever possible. For example, scramble an egg with oil rather than with margarine, and sauté vegetables in oil.

- Select a commercial salad dressing made with a healthy oil. Read the ingredients lists; most dressings are made with soybean oil. To cut calories, choose a low-fat, light, reduced-calorie, or fat-free salad dressing that has a taste you enjoy. Better yet, make your own salad dressing with a healthy oil. By doing this, you can have salad dressings that are much lower in sodium. Whatever salad dressing you use, pour cautiously (or make your own; see p. 40 in chapter 4).

omega-3 fats are canola oil, soybean oil, flax oil, flaxseed, walnut oil, and walnuts. Omega-3 fats are also contained in some fattier fish, such as salmon, trout, albacore tuna, and mackerel. Fish contain more polyunsaturated fat in general than red meats and full-fat dairy foods do. The American Diabetes Association recommends that you get your omega-3 fats by eating fish at least two times a week, not from supplements. Studies show supplements have not been effective to prevent or treat cardiovascular events, such as heart attacks and strokes.

Monounsaturated Fats

Monounsaturated fats are good for your heart. The foods and oils that are the best sources of monounsaturated fats are nuts; canola, olive, and peanut oil; olives; and avocados.

Tips for Eating More Monounsaturated Fats

- Stock canola or extra-virgin olive oil in your cupboard. Use them to sauté, cook, and bake.

- Make your own salad dressing with canola or extra-virgin olive oil. Use the type of olive oil you enjoy most; the color has no impact on calories or types of fats. Extra-virgin is more flavorful and contains a higher amount of beneficial phytochemicals than the lighter, not-first-pressed greener olive oils. (More details on making your own dressing can be found on p. 40 in chapter 4.)

- Enjoy a small handful (about 1 ounce) of almonds, pecans, peanuts, pistachios, cashews, or macadamia nuts as a snack. All nuts are good sources of various types of healthy fats. Sprinkle a few nuts onto salads, cooked or dry cereal, or stir-fries.

- Use a slice or two of avocado on a salad. Spread avocado on a sandwich instead of mayonnaise or butter. Garnish casseroles with avocado, or use it to make guacamole.

- Add a few olives to a relish plate or salad, or use them as a garnish.

Unhealthy Fats

Saturated Fats

Foods with saturated fat are mainly those from animal sources. Red meats, poultry, seafood, whole milk, cheese, ice cream, and butter all contain some saturated fat. Some plant-based oils—coconut, palm, and palm kernel oils—contain saturated fats and are used in some processed crackers, cookies, baked goods, and fried snack foods. Check Table 13.3 to see what saturated fats do to your blood lipids.

Tips for Cutting Down on Saturated Fat

- Purchase lean cuts of meat, and trim the visible fat before cooking.
- Take the skin off poultry (either before or after cooking).
- Eat smaller portions (3 ounces cooked) of meat and meat substitutes. Prepare them in low-fat ways.
- Limit the amount of full-fat cheese you eat and buy reduced-fat and part-skim cheeses. See if they satisfy your taste buds.
- Use fat-free and low-fat milk and yogurt. (Fat-free contains the least fat and calories.)
- Try different brands of low-fat, light, or fat-free cream cheese, cottage cheese, mayonnaise, and sour cream. See if any of them satisfy your taste buds.
- Choose heart-healthy liquid oil or tub margarine instead of using butter, shortening, or other solid fats for cooking and eating.
- Limit the amount of coconut, palm, and palm kernel oil you consume. They contain saturated fats and are in processed foods. Check the ingredients lists for these fats.

Trans Fats

Trans fats are found in some processed foods like crackers, cookies, and ready-to-bake biscuits. These trans fats are created through partial hydrogenation, a process that makes fat hard at room temperature and helps food stay fresh on supermarket shelves and in your cupboard. Research has linked trans fats to increased total and LDL cholesterol levels, decreased healthy HDL levels, and, therefore, increased risk of heart disease.

Since 2006, the Food and Drug Administration (FDA) has required that most packaged foods have food labels showing the amount of trans fat they contain. In response, food manufacturers have decreased the amount of partially hydrogenated oils they use. Restaurants have also reduced their use. Sometimes you will still see "partially hydrogenated oil" in the ingredients list, but the food label will state the product has 0 grams of trans fat. This is because products that contain less than 0.5 grams of trans fat are allowed to round down to zero. While the amount is low, you're still better off limiting these foods as much as possible. In 2015,

Tips for Cutting Down on Trans Fats

- Follow the tips for cutting down on saturated fat in this chapter. These tips will help you reduce your trans fats as well.

- Use the food label to check the amount of trans fats in packaged foods. Be aware of the serving size, and keep in mind that manufacturers can list any amount of trans fat below 0.5 grams per serving as zero.

- Read the ingredients lists and try to limit foods that have partially hydrogenated oils among the top few ingredients.

- Choose a tub margarine or spread with little or no trans fat.

- Minimize the amount of fried restaurant foods you eat. The fat used for frying may contain trans fats.

the FDA set a requirement that, by 2018, companies will need to reformulate products without partially hydrogenated oils and/or petition the FDA to permit their use in specific products.

Total Fat

You may find that you need to work on both the amount and the type of fat you eat. Or maybe you don't eat too much fat, but you need to work on choosing healthier fats. The good news is that when you eat less total fat, you will likely also lower the amount of saturated and trans fats and cholesterol you eat.

Cholesterol Facts

Cholesterol is actually not a fat. In fact, two foods that are very high in cholesterol—liver and shrimp—are very low in fat. Although it may not seem like it, foods that are high in saturated fat are not necessarily high in cholesterol. There's minimal difference between the cholesterol counts of lean meats and higher-fat meats. Cholesterol is discussed with fats because it is a fat-like substance that raises blood cholesterol. Diabetes guidelines encourage you to

Tips to Reduce Total Fat Intake

If you think you are getting more than 35% of your calories from fat or are simply getting too many calories, try these tips:

- Use less butter, margarine, oil, salad dressing, mayonnaise, cheese, cream cheese, and sour cream. Take advantage of the reduced-fat and low-fat versions of foods.
- Eat fried foods only once in a while (less than once a month).
- Prepare foods using low-fat methods: broiling, baking, braising, barbecuing, grilling, poaching, sautéing, and steaming.

Tips to Cut Down on Cholesterol

- Eat smaller portions of red meat, poultry, and seafood.
- Choose reduced-fat and part-skim cheeses.
- Choose low-fat or fat-free milk and yogurt.
- Limit egg yolks to no more than three a week. Use egg whites or egg substitutes instead, or use a combination of one whole egg and one egg white when you make scrambled eggs or omelets.
- Limit foods that are high in cholesterol, such as organ meats and shellfish.
- Eat more plant-based protein foods.

eat no more than 300 milligrams (mg) of cholesterol daily; however, the more recently published 2015–2020 Dietary Guidelines suggest cholesteral is no longer a nutrient of concern and there is no set amount. Dietary cholesterol is found only in foods from animal sources: red meats, organ meats, poultry, seafood, egg yolks, and whole-milk dairy foods.

Tips for Slimming Down Your Favorite Recipes

Use the knowledge you've gained about eating less fat to slim down your favorite recipes and continue to enjoy them. What about Aunt Sally's macaroni and cheese recipe or Grandma Betty's apple cobbler? You may long for them, but they may be high in fat and calories from full-fat dairy foods, fats, and sweeteners.

- **Think of a recipe as a starting point.** Change it any way you want to make it tastier and healthier. For example, you might use a healthy oil rather than butter or margarine to sauté, use less oil to sauté, or add a few drizzles of cooking wine or sherry to add flavor without extra fat. You could raise the fiber level of a meatloaf by adding bulgur or whole-wheat bread, lower the saturated fat content by substituting ground turkey for one-third of the meat, or increase the omega-3 content by adding a few teaspoons of ground flax. Increase the calcium content of an omelet by adding a tablespoon of nonfat dry milk to the egg mixture, and coat the pan with a healthy oil instead of butter or margarine.

- **It is easier to slim down recipes when you cook than when you bake.** You cannot make big changes in recipes for some baked items, such as chocolate cake or sponge cake, because there is a delicate chemistry between ingredients. In some fruit bread, pudding, cheesecake, and other recipes, however, you can cut the sugar by up to one-third and, if you need it to be sweeter, replace the sweetness with a low-calorie sweetener (sugar substitute) that can withstand heat.

- **Baked items that contain fruit, such as fruit cobbler, banana bread, carrot cake, or applesauce cake, will slim down, because fruit provides both sweetness and bulk (volume) to the recipe.**

- **Lower the fat and calorie count of a pie by using a single bottom crust rather than top and bottom crusts.**

- **Look for similar recipes in low-calorie or diabetes cookbooks. Adapt your recipe or try theirs.**

- **When you use less fat, you must add back flavor.** For flavor, add fat-free seasonings, spices, or herbs. Try new ones for new taste treats.

- **Use more or less of an ingredient.** For example, in a recipe for stir-fry, use less protein. Replace the volume with larger quantities of the vegetables in the recipe, or add another vegetable, starch, or fruit. For instance, add pineapple chunks and bean sprouts. A few drops of a spicy hot oil add flavor with few calories.

- **In a meat sauce, use less meat and add more vegetables.** Sauté onions, peppers, mushrooms, and zucchini to add volume to the tomato sauce. In lasagna, use less meat and add a layer of spinach sautéed with a bit of oil and lots of garlic.

- **Substitute an ingredient with more flavor, such as extra-sharp cheese, so you can use less of it.** Or take advantage of lean but flavorful turkey sausage instead of using a larger amount of ground meat in a chili or soup.

- **Drain and pat dry ground meat, bacon, or sausage to get out as much excess fat as you can, and use a smaller amount.**

- **Sauté with less oil or butter than the recipe calls for.** You might need to use a lower heat than suggested to avoid burning the food.

- **Skip the butter or margarine that is often called for in store-bought rice and grain mixtures.** They cook up just fine without it.

- **Take advantage of reduced-fat and reduced-calorie ingredients in some recipes.** For example, you might want to top a Mexican dish with light or fat-free sour cream, make a dip with a combination of fat-free yogurt and light sour cream, or use light cream cheese to make a flavorful spread. Be careful when cooking or baking with these ingredients. When you melt margarine-like spreads that list water as the first ingredient, the water separates from the oil and splatters. These spreads can also alter the texture of baked goods.

- **Use fresh herbs.** You can find them in the supermarket, but buy them no more than a few days before you cook so that they are fresh. If you do not use the fresh herb immediately, wrap it in a slightly damp paper towel, place it in a plastic bag, and use it within a few days. A less expensive way to have fresh herbs is to grow them in a garden or pots. If your recipe calls for dried herbs, use three times the amount of the fresh herb.

- **Buy dried herbs and spices in small quantities because they lose taste over time.** If a recipe calls for fresh herbs, use only one-third of that amount in dried herbs.

• **Check out recipe resources.** The Internet is loaded with recipes. A good place to start is www.diabetes.org. Then search
diabetes or healthy recipes. You'll find more than you'll ever
be able to cook. Borrow low-calorie and diabetes cookbooks
and magazines from the library. Learn healthier ways of cooking and baking, and gather recipes from television cooking
shows or online videos.

TABLE 13.2 Serving Sizes, Calories, and Nutrients for Fats

Food	Serving Size
MONOUNSATURATED FATS	
Almond butter, plain	1 1/2 tsp
Almond milk	1 cup
Almonds, dry-roasted	6 almonds
Avocado	2 Tbsp
Brazil nuts	2 nuts
Cashew butter, plain	1 1/2 tsp
Cashews, salted	6 cashews
Hazelnuts (filberts)	5 nuts
Macadamia nuts, dry-roasted, no-salt-added	3 nuts
Nuts, mixed	6 nuts
Oil, canola	1 tsp
Oil, olive	1 tsp
Oil, peanut	1 tsp
Olives, green, stuffed, large	10 olives
Olives, ripe (black), pitted	8 large
Peanut butter	1 1/2 tsp
Peanuts, dry-roasted, no-salt-added	10 peanuts
Pecans, dry-roasted	4 pecan halves
Pistachios	16 kernels
Spread, plant stanol ester-type: Light	1 Tbsp
Regular	2 tsp
POLYUNSATURATED FATS	
Flaxseed, whole	1 Tbsp
Margarine, liquid, regular	1 tsp
Margarine, regular, stick (65–80% vegetable oil)	1 tsp
Margarine, tub (60–70% vegetable oil)	1 tsp

Calories	Fat (g)	Sat. Fat (g)	Mono-unsat. Fat (g)	Poly-unsat. Fat (g)	Cholesterol (mg)
45	4.3	0.4	2.8	0.9	0
30	2.0	0.0			0
48	4.2	0.3	2.7	1.0	0
45	4.1	0.6	2.7	0.5	0
66	6.6	1.5	2.5	2.1	0
43	3.6	0.6	2.3	0.7	0
52	4.2	1.0	2.5	0.7	0
45	4.4	0.3	3.3	0.6	0
56	5.9	0.9	4.6	0.1	0
37	3.4	1.0	1.9	0.8	0
40	4.5	0.3	2.7	1.3	0
40	4.5	0.6	3.3	0.5	0
40	4.5	0.8	2.1	1.4	0
62	5.0	1.2	3.8	0.5	0
40	3.8	0.5	2.8	0.3	0
48	4.2	0.8	2.0	1.2	0
58	5.0	0.7	2.5	1.6	0
40	4.2	0.4	2.5	1.2	0
64	5.1	0.6	2.7	1.6	0
50	5.0	0.7			0
45	5.0	0.6			0
55	4.3	0.4	0.8	3.0	0
34	3.8	0.5	0.8	2.3	0
30	3.3	0.7	0.9	1.0	0
24	2.7	0.6	0.9	1.1	0

continued

TABLE 13.2 *continued*

Food	Serving Size
Margarine-like spread, tub, light or lower-fat (30–50% vegetable oil)	1 Tbsp
Mayonnaise	1 tsp
Mayonnaise, light (reduced-fat)	1 Tbsp
Mayonnaise-style salad dressing	2 tsp
Mayonnaise-style salad dressing, light	1 Tbsp
Oil, corn	1 tsp
Oil, cottonseed	1 tsp
Oil, flaxseed	1 tsp
Oil, grapeseed	1 tsp
Oil, safflower	1 tsp
Oil, soybean	1 tsp
Oil, soybean and canola (Enova)	1 tsp
Oil, sunflower	1 tsp
Pine nuts (pignolias), dried	1 Tbsp
Pumpkin seeds, roasted	1 Tbsp
Salad dressing, reduced-fat, cream-based	2 Tbsp
Salad dressing, regular	1 Tbsp
Sesame seeds	1 Tbsp
Spread, plant stanol ester, light (Benecol)	1 Tbsp
Spread, plant stanol ester, regular (Benecol)	2 tsp
Sunflower seeds, dry-roasted	1 Tbsp
Tahini (sesame butter or paste)	2 tsp
Walnuts, English, shelled	4 halves
SATURATED FATS	
Bacon grease	1 tsp
Bacon, fried, drained	1 slice (16 per lb)
Bacon, turkey	1 slice
Butter	1 tsp
Butter, light (Land O'Lakes)	1 Tbsp

Calories	Fat (g)	Sat. Fat (g)	Mono-unsat. Fat (g)	Poly-unsat. Fat (g)	Cholesterol (mg)
46	5.0	1.1	1.5	2.3	0
33	3.6	0.5	0.9	2.0	2
45	4.6	0.7	1.1	2.5	4
27	2.3	0.3	0.7	1.3	3
25	1.5	0.3	0.2	1.0	4
40	4.5	0.6	1.2	2.5	0
40	4.5	1.2	0.8	2.3	0
40	4.5	0.4	0.9	3.0	0
40	4.5	0.4	0.7	3.1	0
40	4.5	0.3	0.6	3.4	0
40	4.5	0.6	1.0	2.6	0
40	4.7	0.2	1.7	2.3	0
40	4.5	0.5	0.9	3.0	0
58	5.9	0.4	1.6	2.9	0
73	5.9	1.1	1.8	2.7	0
70	4.0	0.3	1.8	1.5	0
69	6.7	0.8	1.3	3.2	0
52	4.5	0.6	1.7	2.0	0
50	5.0	0.5	2.5	2.0	0
47	5.0	0.3	1.7	1.3	0
47	4.0	0.4	0.8	2.6	0
60	5.4	0.8	2.0	2.4	0
52	5.2	0.5	0.7	3.8	0
39	4.3	2.0	1.9	0.5	4
43	3.3	1.1	1.5	0.4	9
31	2.2	0.7	0.9	0.5	8
38	2.4	0.0	10.0	1.0	27
50	6.0	3.5	1.5	0.0	15

continued

TABLE 13.2 *continued*

Food	Serving Size
Butter, whipped	2 tsp
Butter blends with oil, light	1 Tbsp
Butter blends with oil, regular	1 1/2 tsp
Chitterlings, boiled	2 Tbsp (1/2 oz)
Coconut milk, light	1/3 cup
Coconut milk, regular	1 1/2 Tbsp
Coconut, shredded, dried, sweetened	2 Tbsp
Cream cheese	1 Tbsp (1/2 oz)
Cream cheese, reduced-fat (Neufchâtel)	1 1/2 Tbsp (3/4 oz)
Cream, half & half	2 Tbsp
Cream, heavy (whipping) unwhipped	1 Tbsp
Cream, light	1 1/2 Tbsp
Lard, pork	1 tsp
Oil, coconut	1 tsp
Oil, palm	1 tsp
Oil, palm kernel	1 tsp
Salt pork, fresh, cooked	1/4 oz
Shortening	1 tsp
Sour cream, reduced-fat or light	3 Tbsp
Sour cream, regular	2 Tbsp
Whipped cream, pressurized, regular	1/4 cup
Whipped cream, sweetened	2 Tbsp

Source: Adapted from *Choose Your Foods: Food Lists for Diabetes.* Academy of Nutrition and Dietetics and American Diabetes Association, 2014.

Calories	Fat (g)	Sat. Fat (g)	Mono-unsat. Fat (g)	Poly-unsat. Fat (g)	Cholesterol (mg)
33	4.0	2.3	1.4	0.2	10
50	5.0	2.0	–	–	5
50	5.5	2.2	–	–	10
38	3.3	1.5	1.1	0.2	44
47	4.0	2.7	0.7	0.1	0
44	4.8	4.3	0.2	0.1	0
42	2.6	2.4	0.1	0.0	0
51	4.6	3.1	1.4	0.2	20
54	4.6	3.1	1.5	0.2	15
39	3.5	2.1	1.0	0.1	11
52	5.5	3.5	1.6	0.2	21
44	4.3	2.7	1.3	0.2	15
39	4.3	1.7	1.9	0.5	4
39	4.5	3.9	0.3	0.1	0
40	4.5	2.2	1.7	0.4	0
39	4.5	3.7	0.5	0.1	0
51	5.4	1.9	2.6	0.6	6
38	4.3	1.1	1.9	1.1	0
61	3.7	3.0	0.6	0.2	18
62	4.8	3.4	1.4	0.1	19
39	3.3	2.1	1.0	0.1	11
52	5.2	3.2	1.5	0.2	19

CHAPTER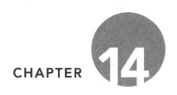

Sweets, Desserts, and Other Sugary Foods

What's Ahead?

→ Types of sugary foods and sweets in this food group.
→ The nutrition drawbacks of sugary foods and sweets (hint: there are no benefits).
→ Healthy eating goals for sugary foods and sweets.
→ Assess the servings of the sugary foods and sweets you eat.
→ All about sugar alcohols, sugar substitutes, and so-called sugar-free foods.
→ Tips to help you limit sugary foods and sweets.
→ Serving sizes and nutrition numbers for sugary foods and sweets.

Sugary Foods, Sweets, and Diabetes

Good news! People with diabetes are no longer being told sugary foods and sweets are forbidden. The American Diabetes Association revised their recommendation about axing sugary foods and sweets in 1994, over two decades ago. Today's recommendations continue to point out that similar amounts of carbohydrate from all sources of carbohydrate (bread, pasta, fruit, or sugar from sweets) raise blood glucose levels similarly.

Blood glucose management is one reason to eat fewer sugary foods and sweets, but your health and weight are two others. The recommendation to eat sugary foods and sweets in moderation is the same as for the general public. One reason to limit sugary foods and sweets is that they're concentrated sources of calories. Because most people with prediabetes or type 2 diabetes need to lose weight, limiting calories from sugary foods and sweets can be helpful. There just isn't much calorie wiggle room for these foods. With regard to sugar-sweetened beverages, the American Diabetes Association now recommends that people with diabetes limit or avoid them to reduce the risk of weight gain and worsening of cardiovascular risk factors.

Table 14.1 at the end of this chapter (starting on page 210) shows the serving sizes for sugary foods and sweets, along with information on calories, carbohydrate, total fat, saturated fat, and cholesterol content.

What Are "Sugars"?

Notice the use of the term "sugars" instead of "sugar." The term "sugars" doesn't just include the white granulated stuff we keep in that bowl on our table or in our pantry to use in baking. The term "sugars" more accurately describes these two types of sugars in foods:

- **Naturally occurring sugars:** Some healthy foods contain naturally occurring sugars, which provide healthy sources of energy, carbohydrate, vitamins, and minerals. Examples include sucrose and fructose in fruit and lactose in milk.

- **Added sugars:** The sugars are added to foods during food processing, in food preparation, or at the table. The added sugars used in food manufacturing, particularly sugar-sweetened beverages, are now the greatest contributor of sugars to our diet. Today, the added sugar used most commonly in manufactured foods and beverages is high fructose corn syrup. While there's been a lot of research and discussion about high fructose corn syrup, the American Diabetes Association nutrition recommendations suggest that the relatively minimal amount of this form of fructose that most people consume is not likely to have a detrimental effect on triglycerides (the form of fat that travels in our blood and one of the blood lipid measures).

All sugars, from natural sources or added, contain 4 calories per gram because they are 100% carbohydrate. Knowing the names of the different sugars out there helps you make healthy decisions when you read Nutrition Facts labels (see the list on page 203).

What Are "Sugary Foods"?

"Sugary foods" are foods that contain added sugars but aren't considered a dessert. They include jams, jellies, and sweetened yogurt; condiments such as salad dressings and ketchup; and sauces like barbecue, plum, and sweet-and-sour. If you have diabetes, be mindful of these stealthy sugars. For example, you may find that Asian foods can wreak havoc with your blood glucose. This shouldn't be a surprise because many Asian dishes use sugar in marinades and sauces and cornstarch to thicken sauces.

What Are Sweets?

Sweets and desserts typically contain added sugars and often fats. They include cake, cookies, and ice cream. You may not realize that it's the fats in most sweets, not the sugars, that raise the calorie count. In addition, many sweets contain saturated and trans fats and cholesterol, depending on the ingredients used to make the sweets. If a sweet contains butter and eggs, it will contain cholesterol. If it contains partially hydrogenated oils, it will contain trans fats.

If you need to lose weight or if your blood fats aren't under control, particularly triglycerides, you may need to cut back on sweets. Table 14.2 shows how the calories mount up when fat creeps into sweets.

Sugary Foods and Sweets: Just How Much?

High intake of added sugars is one of the greatest nutritional concerns today. Our intake has risen steadily over the last 20 years. Health experts believe that our added sugars consumption is a big contributor to the twin epidemics of obesity and type 2 diabetes, as well as a big reason people don't eat enough nutrient-dense foods. The calories from these foods and drinks crowd the healthier foods and calories out of our diets.

It's not that sugars or sugary foods cause diabetes. We know that's not true, but all these extra calories can certainly contribute to weight gain over the years.

Americans eat an estimated 17 teaspoons of added sugars every day! This may seem hard to believe, but consider that a 20-ounce regularly sweetened soft drink contains about 15 teaspoons of added sugars (and we know they come in much bigger servings). It seems much more believable now, doesn't it? Beyond sugar-sweet-

TABLE 14.2	Nutritional Value of Some Sweets and Desserts with and without Added Fat			
Food	Serving	Calories	Carb (g)	Fat (g)
Strawberry gelatin (regular)	1/2 cup	70	15	0
Strawberry pie (two-crust)	*1 serving*	*360*	*49*	*18*
Chocolate chips	1 Tbsp	66	9	4
Chocolate chip cookies	*2 small*	*248*	*28*	*14*
Jelly beans	10 (1 oz)	66	26	0
Lemon meringue pie	1 piece	362	49	16
Sugar, granulated	1 Tbsp	48	12	0
Ice cream (regular, store brand)	1/2 cup	132	16	7
Ice cream (premium)	*1/2 cup*	*280*	*20*	*20*

Entries in italics include added fats.

ened beverages, which contribute over one-third of the added sugars we take in daily, our other large sources of added sugars are in candy and grain-based desserts like cakes, cookies, pies, and pastries. Dairy-based desserts like ice cream are another significant source of added sugars.

The recommendations for healthy eating suggest that you eat no more than a few teaspoons of added sugars a day. People who need to reduce their caloric intake each day to lose or maintain a healthy weight can't "afford" many calories for sugary foods and sweets. People who can eat more calories because they are at a healthy weight, are larger in stature, or burn a lot of calories due to physical activity can allot more calories for sugary foods and sweets. Table 14.3 applies these guidelines to the calorie ranges in this book.

Get to Know Yourself

If you want to change your eating habits, you need to take stock of your current eating habits. Ask yourself these questions about the sugary foods and sweets you eat.

- Which foods and beverages do I add sugars to during preparation or while eating?

- Which foods do I eat that contain added sugars? How often and in what quantity do I eat these foods?

- Do I often drink beverages that contain added sugars?

TABLE 14.3	Daily Recommendation for Added Sugars
Calorie Range	Added Sugars (tsp)
1,200–1,400	4
1,400–1,600	4
1,600–1,900	4–7
1,900–2,300	8–11
2,300–2,800	12–18

- Do I use sugar substitutes?

- How many times a day or a week do I eat sweets (desserts)?

- What are my favorite sweets?

- How often can I or do I want to fit them into my healthy eating plan?

Total Carbohydrate, Sugars, and the Nutrition Facts Label

When you pick up a food and review the current Nutrition Facts label, you may zero in on the sugars because you think they deserve the most attention. That's not true. Look at this Nutrition Facts label for fat-free milk and you'll notice "Sugars" indented under the bold "Total Carbohydrate." The grams of Sugars are accounted for within the grams of Total Carbohydrate. The grams of sugars in a food are a total of both the natural and the added sugars in one serving.

The term "sugars," according to the current Food and Drug Administration (FDA) definition, includes all the one- and two-unit sugars. A one-unit sugar is glucose or fructose. A two-unit sugar is sucrose, made up of glucose and fructose, or lactose, made up of galactose and glucose. Two-unit sugars are common in some foods, such as fruit and milk. The Nutrition Facts label shows that there are 14 grams of sugars and 14 grams of total carbohydrate in one serving of fat-free milk. Sugars account for all of the carbohydrate in the milk. Does milk have added sugar? No, the sugars are the natural milk sugars—lactose.

The Nutrition Facts label doesn't currently tell you whether the sugars are from natural or added sources, although that may well

Nutrition Facts	
Serving Size 8 fl oz (240mL) Servings Per Container 8	
Amount Per Serving	
Calories 90	Calories from Fat 0
	% Daily Value*
Total Fat 0g	0%
Saturated Fat 0g	0%
Trans Fat 0g	
Cholesterol 5mg	2%
Sodium 120mg	5%
Total Carbohydrate 14g	5%
Dietary Fiber 0g	0%
Sugars 14g	
Protein 9g	
Vitamin A 10% • Vitamin C 0%	
Calcium 35% • Iron 0%	
Vitamin D 25%	

*Percent Daily Values are based on a 2,000 calorie diet. Your daily values may be higher or lower depending on your calorie needs:

		Calories:	2,000	2,500
Total Fat	Less than		65g	80g
Saturated Fat	Less than		20g	25g
Cholesterol	Less than		300mg	300mg
Sodium	Less than		2,400mg	2,400mg
Total Carbohydrate			300g	375g
Dietary Fiber			25g	30g

Calories per gram:
Fat 9 • Carbohydrate 4 • Protein 4

change as the Nutrition Facts label is updated in the near future. In fact, the FDA, in their proposal for a new nutrition label, wants to require information about added sugars in addition to naturally occurring sugars. The FDA has also proposed including a percent Daily Value for added sugars on the Nutrition Facts label, with the recommendation that the daily intake from added sugars not exceed 10% of total calories. While waiting for the new nutrition facts label, gain insight into the sources of sugars in a food by reading the ingredient list (ingredients used in the product are listed in descending order by weight). You might also see these words, which also mean added sugars: "corn sweetener," "corn syrup," "fruit juice concentrate," "high fructose corn syrup," "dextrose," "glucose," "maltose," "sucrose," "honey," molasses, "agave syrup," "raw sugar," "syrup," "malt sugar," or "malt syrup."

Fructose, Honey, and Other "More Natural" Sweeteners

Are fructose, honey, agave nectar, and evaporated cane juice better for you than sugar? No. Fructose, honey, fruit juice concentrates, and other sweeteners raise blood glucose just like other sugars. One is no healthier than another. They have about the same number of calories and, other than fructose (this is not high fructose corn syrup, which contains about half fructose and half glucose), raise blood glucose at about the same speed. Fructose does raise blood glucose more slowly, but in large quantities it may impact your blood lipids.

Reduced-Calorie Sweeteners

There are two main groups of reduced-calorie sweeteners used in sugar-free foods today.

1. Sugar substitutes or no-calorie sweeteners (also called non-nutritive sweeteners or low-calorie sweeteners).

2. Polyols, also called sugar alcohols.

Sugar Substitutes

First, a bit of terminology. Several terms are used to describe this category of sweeteners. The terms "sugar substitute," "low-" or "no-calorie sweeteners," and "artificial sweeteners" are synonymous.

Today there are seven low-calorie sweeteners that have been approved through the FDA's food additive approval process. Several others have been approved through another FDA process called GRAS (Generally Recognized as Safe): a group of stevia-based sweeteners (steviol glycosides), luo han guo (monk fruit), and allulose, a corn-based sweetener. Steviol glycosides are highly purified forms of certain parts of the stevia plant. (This is not the same product as the stevia sold as a dietary supplement.)

All of these sugar substitutes have undergone lengthy safety research and reviews and have been shown to be safe for everyone, including people with diabetes, pregnant and breast-feeding women, and children.

The low-calorie sweeteners approved as food additives are:

- Acesulfame potassium
- Advantame
- Allulose
- Aspartame
- Neotame
- Saccharin
- Sucralose

The main low-calorie sweeteners in use today are acesulfame potassium, aspartame, saccharin, and sucralose. They are used singly or in combination in some foods and beverages, including diet sodas, fruit drinks, syrups, yogurts, ice cream, jams, and other products. They are also available in packets or as granulated products to use like sugar for sweetening foods or for cooking and baking. The sweeteners contain almost no calories or carbohydrate, and they don't raise blood glucose. The packets and granular products do contain a few calories contributed by carbohydrate-based bulking ingredients such as dextrose and maltodextrin.

TABLE 14.4	Comparison of Fruit Drink with Regular and No-Calorie Sweeteners			
Type of Drink	Serving Size	Calories	Carbohydrate (g)	Sugars (g)
Regularly sweetened fruit drink	8 ounces	110	30	29
No-calorie fruit drink	8 ounces	10	2	0

Sugar substitutes can help you greatly lower the carbohydrates and calories you eat. Table 14.4 has a comparison between a regularly sweetened fruit drink and a fruit drink sweetened with a no-caloric sweetener.

Polyols (Sugar Alcohols)

Sugar alcohols (polyols) are a group of ingredients commonly used in sugar-free foods. Interestingly, they're not sugar or alcohol. Rather, they are carbohydrate-based ingredients that contain, on average, half the calories of sugars (2 calories versus 4 calories per gram). Polyols can replace sugar in foods such as candy, cookies, and ice creams.

Common names are "isomalt," "sorbitol," "lactitol," "maltitol," "mannitol," and "xylitol." Note the common "-ol" ending. Polyols contain about half the calories of sugar because they aren't completely digested. A downside of polyols is that in large amounts they may cause gas, cramps, or diarrhea. Some people, especially children, may be bothered by this side effect. Foods that contain larger amounts of polyols must contain an FDA-required statement on the label about this possible "laxative effect."

Replacing sugars with polyols in a food can cause a lower rise in blood glucose than regularly sweetened foods; however, people don't tend to use these foods frequently enough to result in a significant reduction of calorie intake, carbohydrate intake, or blood glucose. The calories and grams of carbohydrate per serving of sugar-free foods sweetened with polyols often are only minimally

TABLE 14.5	Comparison of Ice Cream with Regular and Sugar Alcohol Sweeteners						
Type of Ice Cream	Serving Size	Calories	Total Fat (g)	Carbohydrate (g)	Sugars (g)	Sugar Alcohol (g)
Regular	1/2 cup	140	8	15	15	0
No sugar-added, light	1/2 cup	100	5	15	4	3

reduced. Table 14.5 has a comparison of regular ice cream and ice cream sweetened with a sugar alcohol.

BLENDS OF ADDED SUGARS AND REDUCED-CALORIE SWEETENERS.

The availability of more polyols and no-calorie sweeteners has allowed food manufacturers to create a wider variety of sugar-free and lower-sugar foods. Some examples are calorie-free diet sodas sweetened with one or more no-calorie sweeteners, sugar-free ice cream sweetened with a low-calorie sweetener and one or more polyols, and blended sweeteners for baking that combine sugar and a no-calorie sweetener. Before you buy a product, read the ingredients list to find out which sweeteners are used.

Sugar-Free Foods

If you use foods with polyols or no-calorie sweeteners, read the ingredients and review the Nutrition Facts label to figure out how to fit these foods into your healthy eating plan. Some of these foods can help you satisfy your sweet tooth without putting you over the top of your added sugars count. According to the American Diabetes Association, it is not necessary to subtract the grams of sugar alcohols in foods from your total carbohydrate count because the amounts are neglible and inconsequential.

The "Sugar-Free" Nutrition Claim

Foods and beverages labeled "sugar-free," or alternatively "no sugar added," aren't necessarily carbohydrate- or calorie-free. The calorie count depends on which sweeteners (added sugars, polyols, or sugar substitutes) have been used in the food as well as the other ingredients. Remember, according to the FDA's definition, "sugars" are defined as all one- and two-unit sugars. The calorie-containing sweetening ingredients in some sugar-free foods, such as sorbitol and mannitol, aren't "sugars" by the FDA definition, but they still contain carbohydrate and calories. The sugar substitutes in some sugar-free foods don't contain calories or carbohydrate. Whether sugar-free foods cause a rise in blood glucose depends on the sweeteners and other ingredients in the food.

There is no doubt that many sugar-free foods—especially those sweetened with low-calorie sweeteners, such as diet carbonated and noncarbonated drinks, hot cocoa, yogurt, and syrups—can help satisfy your sweet tooth, reduce your waistline, lower your blood glucose, and perhaps improve your blood lipids (as long as you consume them as part of an otherwise healthy lifestyle). Explore a variety of sugar-free foods. Find a few that truly offer you a calorie savings and help you stay on track with your nutrition and diabetes goals.

Fitting in Sugars and Sweets

When you choose to eat sugary foods or sweets, substitute them for other carbohydrate in your eating plan, or burn more calories. Consider these questions when you decide how many sugary foods and sweets to eat.

- Are my blood glucose and A1C on target or higher than desirable?

- Are my blood lipids (LDL, HDL, and triglycerides) in the target range?

- Do I need to lose weight, which means that I cannot afford a lot of calories in the form of sugary foods and sweets?

- How much do I enjoy sugary foods and sweets, and how often do I feel I need to have a small serving to stay on track and be satisfied?

- How can I best control portion sizes of sugars and sweets?

- Can I be more physically active after eating sugary foods and sweets so I can burn the extra calories that come from them?

Tips for Minimizing Added Sugars and Sweets

- Prioritize your personal diabetes goals. Which is most critical for you: keeping your blood glucose levels on target, losing weight, or lowering your blood lipids? Your priorities should dictate how you strike the balance with sugary foods and sweets.

- Choose a few favorite desserts and decide how often to eat them in light of your personal diabetes goals: maybe twice a week, just when dining out, or only at a special celebration.

- Note the calories, total fat, saturated fat, and cholesterol of the desserts you prefer. Then make your choices with these numbers and your diabetes goals in mind.

- Satisfy your sweet tooth with a small portion of your favorite sweet. Don't waste your calories on just-so-so sweets.

- Split desserts (at least in half) when you eat out.

- Take advantage of smaller portions when you can (child-size or one-scoop servings for ice cream).

- Use the Nutrition Facts label to see how many grams of carbohydrate there are per serving. You need this information to swap a sweet food for other carbohydrate in your meal plan.

- Check the Nutrition Facts label for the grams of sugars under Total Carbohydrate, and read the ingredients list to try to decipher which natural and added sugars are present.

- When you eat a sweet, check your blood glucose 1–2 hours afterward to see its effect. You might find that the same quantity of ice cream raises your blood glucose more slowly than frozen yogurt, which contains less fat and more carbohydrate. Let this information help you decide which sweets to eat, when to eat them, and how much to eat.

- Explore sugar-free options. With some foods, such as diet drinks and coffee sweeteners, it's a no-brainer and can save you a boatload of calories. Learn to cook and bake with a no-calorie sweetener. Find a few foods that truly save calories and satisfy your sweet tooth.

TABLE 14.1	Serving Sizes, Calories, and Nutrients for Sugary Foods and Sweets

Food	Serving Size
BEVERAGES, SODAS, AND ENERGY/SPORTS DRINKS	
Cranberry juice cocktail	1/2 cup
Energy drink	1 can (8.3 fl oz)
Fruit punch drink	1 cup (8 fl oz)
Hot chocolate (cocoa)	1 envelope (0.7 oz)
Hot chocolate (cocoa), sugar-free	1 envelope (0.53 oz)
Hot cocoa mix, lite	1 envelope (0.75 oz)
Lemonade, prepared	1 cup (8 fl oz)
Soft drink (soda), regular	1 can (12 fl oz)
Sports drink	1 cup
BROWNIES, CAKE, COOKIES, GELATIN, PIE, AND PUDDING	
Angel food cake, unfrosted	1 slice (about 2 oz)
Biscotti	1 oz
Brownie, small, unfrosted	1 brownie (1 1/4" sq, 7/8" high)
Cake, frosted	1 square (2")
Cake, unfrosted	1 square (2")
Cookies, 100-calorie pack	1 oz
Cookies, chocolate chip	2 cookies, medium (2 1/4" dia)
Cookies, gingersnap, regular	3 cookies
Cookies, sandwich, cream filling	2 cookies, small
Cookies, sugar-free	3 cookies, small
Cookies, vanilla wafers	5 wafers
Cupcake, small, frosted	1 cupcake, small
Flan	1/2 cup
Fruit cobbler	1/2 cup
Gelatin, regular	1/2 cup
Pie, fruit, 2-crust	1 slice (1/6th pie)
Pie, pumpkin or custard	1 slice (1/8th pie)

Calories (g)	Carbohydrate (g)	Fat (g)	Saturated Fat (g)	Cholesterol (mg)
68	17.1	0.1	0.0	0
125	32.5	0.2	0.0	0
97	4.8	0.0	0.0	0
80	15.0	3.0	2.0	0
50	9.9	0.4	0.1	1
80	7.0	1.0	0.0	0
112	28.7	0.0	0.0	0
147	37.6	0.0	0.0	0
50	14.0	0.0	0.0	0
128	29.4	0.2	0.0	0
130	17.0	6.0	1.0	10
115	18.1	4.6	1.2	5
175	29.2	6.4	2.0	18
97	16.6	3.1	1.0	18
110	22.0	3.5	0.8	0
156	18.7	9.1	2.6	10
87	16.1	2.1	0.5	0
93	14.3	3.8	0.7	0
141	20.4	6.9	1.8	0
88	14.7	3.0	0.8	10
174	29.2	6.1	1.3	8
220	35.0	6.0	2.8	140
84	19.2	0.0	0.0	0
80	19.0	0.0	0.0	0
284	42.4	12.5	2.0	0
168	21.8	7.6	1.4	16

continued

TABLE 14.1 *continued*	
Food	**Serving Size**
Pudding, regular (reduced-fat milk)	1/2 cup
Pudding, sugar-free, fat-free (fat-free milk)	1/2 cup
CANDY, SPREADS, SWEETS, SWEETENERS, SYRUPS, AND TOPPINGS	
Blended sweeteners (mixtures of artificial sweeteners and sugar)	1 1/2 Tbsp
Candy bar, chocolate or peanut-type	2 bars, fun size (1/2 oz each)
Candy, hard	3 pieces
Chocolate, dark- or milk-type	1 oz
Chocolate kisses	5 kisses
Coffee creamer, dry, flavored	4 tsp
Coffee creamer, liquid, flavored	2 Tbsp
Fruit snack (chewy roll)	1 roll
Fruit spread, 100% fruit (jam, preserves)	1 1/2 Tbsp
Honey, strained	1 Tbsp
Jam or preserves, regular	1 Tbsp
Jelly, regular	1 Tbsp
Sugar, white, granulated	1 Tbsp
Syrup, chocolate	2 Tbsp
Syrup, pancake-type, light	2 Tbsp
Syrup, pancake-type, regular	1 Tbsp
CONDIMENTS AND SAUCES	
Barbecue sauce, bottled	3 Tbsp
Cranberry sauce, canned, sugar added	1/4 cup
Gravy, canned or bottled	1/2 cup
Hoisin sauce	1 Tbsp
Marinade	1 Tbsp
Plum sauce	1 Tbsp
Salad dressing, fat-free/low-fat, cream-based	3 Tbsp
Sauce, sweet-and-sour	3 Tbsp

Calories (g)	Carbohydrate (g)	Fat (g)	Saturated Fat (g)	Cholesterol (mg)
141	25.9	2.4	1.4	10
70	11.9	0.2	0.0	2
70	18.0	0.0	0.0	0
151	19.8	7.5	2.6	2
59	14.7	0.0	0.0	0
155	17.0	9.0	5.3	0
105	12.2	6.1	3.7	3
60	9.0	2.3	1.5	0
70	11.0	3.0	0.6	0
78	17.7	1.5	0.0	0
60	15.0	0.0	0.0	0
64	17.3	0.0	0.0	0
48	12.9	0.0	0.0	0
52	13.4	0.0	0.0	0
48	12.5	0.0	0.0	0
109	25.4	0.4	0.2	0
50	13.0	0.0	0.0	0
50	13.2	0.0	0.0	0
79	19.0	0.2	0.0	0
104	26.8	0.1	0.0	0
53	6.4	0.0	0.3	1
35	7.0	0.5	0.1	0
30	6.0	0.0	0.0	0
35	8.0	0.0	0.0	0
63	15.4	0.1	0.0	0
67	16.1	0.0	0.0	0

continued

TABLE 13.1 *continued*	
Food	**Serving Size**
DOUGHNUTS, MUFFINS, PASTRIES, AND SWEET BREADS	
Banana nut bread	1 slice (1" thick)
Danish pastry, fruit-type	1 pastry (4 1/4" dia)
Doughnut, cake-type, plain	1 medium
Doughnut, yeast-type, glazed	1 doughnut (3 3/4" dia)
Muffin	1/4 large
Scone	1 scone (4 oz)
Sweet roll	1 roll
FROZEN BARS, FROZEN DESSERTS, FROZEN YOGURT, AND ICE CREAM	
Frozen pop, juice-type	1 pop
Fruit juice bar, frozen, 100% juice	1 bar (3 oz)
Ice cream	1/2 cup
Ice cream, fat-free	1/2 cup
Ice cream, light	1/2 cup
Ice cream, no-sugar-added	1/2 cup
Sherbet	1/2 cup
Sorbet	1/2 cup
Yogurt, frozen, fat-free	1/3 cup
Yogurt, frozen, regular	1/2 cup
Yogurt, frozen, Greek, lower-fat or fat-free	1/2 cup
GRANOLA BARS, MEAL REPLACEMENT BARS/SHAKES, AND TRAIL MIX	
Granola bar	1 bar (1 oz)
Granola bar, chewy, low-fat	1 bar (1 oz)
Meal replacement bar, medium	1 bar (2 oz)
Meal replacement bar, small	1 bar (1 1/3 oz)
Meal replacement shake, reduced-calorie	1 can (10–11 oz)
Trail mix, candy and nut–based	1 oz
Trail mix, fruit-based	1 oz

Source: Adapted from *Choose Your Foods: Food Lists for Diabetes.* Academy of Nutrition and Dietetics and American Diabetes Association, 2014.

Calories (g)	Carbohydrate (g)	Fat (g)	Saturated Fat (g)	Cholesterol (mg)
178	30.5	5.4	2.2	34
263	33.9	13.1	3.5	81
196	21.4	11.1	3.3	4
239	30.4	11.5	3.3	18
103	12.9	5.0	2.0	16
405	58.0	17.0	8.8	70
264	36.1	11.6	2.2	47
27	6.5	0.1	0.0	0
75	18.6	0.1	0.0	0
165	15.0	10.0	4.5	23
90	22.0	0.0	0.0	0
120	16.0	5.0	2.0	15
115	14.5	5.5	2.3	10
138	29.2	1.9	1.1	0
130	31.2	0.0	0.0	0
66	13.2	0.0	0.0	5
110	18.5	3.3	1.7	10
110	21.0	1.0	0.8	5
134	18.3	5.6	1.0	0
109	21.9	2.0	0.5	0
202	27.0	5.3	3.0	2
140	21.5	4.2	1.8	2
220	38.0	3.0	0.5	5
137	12.7	9.0	1.7	1
115	18.6	4.8	2.4	0

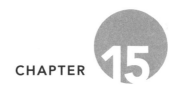

CHAPTER

Beverages: Non Alcoholic

What's Ahead?

→ What the category of non alcoholic beverages includes.
→ Healthier and less-than-healthy beverage options.
→ About added sugars in non alcoholic beverages.
→ Assess your current habits with non alcoholic beverages.
→ Tips to sip by without tanking up on lots of calories.

Non alcoholic beverages don't really constitute a food group, but today people often accumulate more than 500 calories a day sipping their favorite hot or cold beverages. Is this true for you? You may not even be conscious of the calories you drink. They add up fast. If you become aware of what and how much you drink, you can learn to make healthier choices. Selecting healthier no- or low-calorie beverages can be a painless way to cut calories and lose weight, as well as control your blood glucose. You don't have to sip less, just differently!

Today, you can sip calories in many forms, including regularly sweetened soda, fruit drinks, flavored seltzers, fruit juice, sports drinks, energy drinks, hot or iced coffee with syrups and whipped cream, green and chai tea, smoothies, and drinkable yogurt.

Unfortunately, many of these beverages are sweetened with added sugars, which result in loads of calories and grams of carbohydrates with no nutrition and actually some health hazards. Thankfully, there's water and a few other beverages with next to no calories. Table 15.1 shows just some of the healthier alternatives to your favorite regularly sweetened drinks.

TABLE 15.1 Healthier Alternatives to Sweetened Beverages	
Less-Healthy Beverages with Added Sugars	**Healthier Beverages with No Calories**
Soda, regularly sweetened or sweetened with a combination of regular sweeteners and no-calorie sweetener	Mineral, sparkling, or still water; diet soda; club soda; diet tonic water; flavored seltzer water with no-calorie sweetener
Fruit drink, punch, lemonade and other "-ades"	Fruit punch with no-calorie sweetener
Sports drink, regular	Sports drink with no-calorie sweetener
Fruit juice made with 100% juice and fortified*	Fruit punch with no-calorie sweetener; flavored seltzer water with no-calorie sweetener
Coffee, hot or iced, with syrup and whipped cream	Coffee with no-calorie sweetener
Tea with added sugars	Tea with no-calorie sweetener

*Though it is best to eat your fruit as pieces of fresh, canned, frozen, or dried fruit, 100% fruit juice contains many nutrients. If you drink fruit juice, choose one that is fortified with calcium or other nutrients you need. Also, when you do drink fruit juice, measure out the proper portion because it's easy to drink large portions.

Weigh In on Water

Water makes up about 60% of your body weight and is an essential nutrient. A constant supply of water is vital to keep your body functioning properly. Water contains no calories. You can drink as much as you want! You get water from the liquids you drink and the food you eat. Foods like vegetables, fruit, and milk contain a high percentage of water. People need roughly 8 cups (64 ounces) of fluids per day, but the latest guidelines for fluid consumption note that the amount people need varies greatly based on the climate you live in, the type of work you do, and your level of physical activity. Keep yourself properly hydrated, and use your thirst as an indicator of how much water or other liquids you need. Safe tap or bottled water is by far the healthiest beverage for quenching your thirst.

Health Concerns about Beverages with Added Sugars

- The average person consumes about one-third of their added sugars per day from regularly sweetened soda.

- People who drink regularly sweetened beverages are more likely to gain weight and have cardiovascular problems.

- People who eat and drink more added sugars tend to consume more calories, yet they don't get the nutrition they need. They eat insufficient amounts of foods that provide dietary fiber, vitamins, and minerals.

- Calories ingested as liquids may be more likely to cause weight gain than calories eaten as solid foods because you have to take time to chew them. However, the jury is still out on this question.

Get to Know Yourself

If you want to change your habits, you need to take stock of your current drinking habits. Ask yourself these questions about what and how much you drink.

- What beverages do I regularly drink and in what quantities?
- How many calories do the beverages I drink add up to in a day?
- What changes am I willing to make in the beverages I select?

Nutrition Facts Tell the Truth

Don't be led astray with the word "natural," the healthy pictures of fresh fruit on regularly sweetened drinks and drinkable yogurts, or the glowing advertisements about athletic performance on sports drinks. This is mostly hype. To find out what's really in the bottle or can, look to the Nutrition Facts label. Check out the serving size, calories, and carbohydrate. If the drink contains no calories or grams of carbohydrate, then it is probably not sweetened with added sugars. To know for sure, check the ingredients. High fructose corn syrup is the sweetener you find in most regularly sweetened bottled or canned drinks. You might also see the words "corn sweetener," "corn syrup," "fruit juice concentrate," "dextrose," "glucose," or "malt syrup."

Another food-labeling law requires manufacturers to tell you the exact percentage of fruit juice used in a fruit beverage. Manufacturers can only use the term "juice" if the product is 100% fruit juice. A fruit "drink," like many of the products on the supermarket and convenience store shelves today, only has to contain 10% fruit juice. Some of them contain more, but most of these drinks are sweetened with added sugars.

It's Easy to Fill Up on Too Much

Table 15.2 shows how easy it is to fill your tank with a lot of calories and grams of carbohydrate just from one day's worth of beverages.

Table 15.3 shows how changing your beverage choices can make a big dent in your calorie and carbohydrate totals.

In total, the change would mean a whopping 624 fewer calories and 141 fewer grams of carbohydrate. And it's a simple and easy way to reduce your intake!

TABLE 15.2 **Calories in Regular Beverages**

Name of drink	Amount	Calories	Carb (g)
Orange juice	12 ounces	164	38
Milk, whole	8 ounces	150	12
Soda, regular	20-ounce bottle	258	66
Sports drink, regular	16-ounce bottle	112	28
Coffee frappe, blended coffee drink	16 ounces	260	52
Total		944	196

TABLE 15.3 **Lower-Calorie Beverage Options**

Name of drink	Amount	Calories	Carb (g)
Orange juice	8 ounces	110	25
Milk, fat-free	8 ounces	90	12
Soda, diet	20-ounce bottle	0	0
Sports drink, sweetened with no-calorie sweetener	16-ounce bottle	20	4
Cappuccino, sweetened with fat-free milk	16 ounces	100	14
Total		320	55

Healthier Ways to Quench Your Thirst

Instead of reaching for a beverage sweetened with added sugars, try these healthy tips:

- Quench your thirst with water. In most places, tap water is safe, healthy, and tasty.

- If you tire of water, choose club soda, seltzer, or sparkling water. To give water or these other drinks a new flavor at home or in restaurants, squeeze in a splash of fresh lemon, lime, or orange.

- When you choose milk, choose fat-free milk. If you just can't stand fat-free, use no more than 1% milk.

- When you choose juice, make sure it's 100% fruit juice, and limit the amount you drink. If possible, buy 100% juice fortified with calcium or vitamin D.

- Stock your home with healthy drinks only: fat-free milk, fortified 100% juice, and water. Make these the options for meals and snacks for both kids and adults.

- If you choose a drinkable or squeeze yogurt, make sure it's sweetened with a no-calorie sweetener.

- If you drink soda, select a diet soda sweetened with one or more no-calorie sweeteners (sugar substitutes).

- Sweeten your coffee or tea with a no-calorie sweetener.

- If you order a specialty coffee or tea, order it made with fat-free milk. Sweeten it with a no-calorie sweetener.

- When you make iced tea, lemonade, or a dry-powdered fruit drink like Kool-Aid or Crystal Light, sweeten it with a no- or low-calorie sweetener rather than sugar, or buy a ready-made low-calorie drink.

- If you buy a sports drink, iced tea, or fruit drink, make it one sweetened with a no-calorie sweetener.

- When you eat in restaurants, order water, diet soda, 100% fruit juice, or low-fat milk.

CHAPTER

Beverages: Alcoholic

What's Ahead?

→ Definitions of a moderate amount and a serving of alcohol.

→ How to assess your current habits with alcoholic beverages.

→ The upside and downside of drinking alcohol.

→ Why, when, and how people with diabetes should or shouldn't drink alcohol.

→ What to watch for if you drink alcohol and have diabetes.

→ Tips for drinking alcohol safely and responsibly.

Alcoholic beverages don't constitute a food group. You don't need to drink alcohol to eat (and drink) healthfully. However, research shows there are actually a few health benefits to drinking moderate amounts of alcohol, and these benefits may be particularly valuable for people at risk for or with diabetes. On the flip side, alcohol can have some serious drawbacks for people with certain medical conditions or who take certain medications.

Alcohol may not be a food group, but it is a potential source of calories, which many people need to factor into their calorie allotment. Alcohol contains 7 calories per gram, right between the 4 calories per gram of carbohydrate and protein and the 9 of fat. These calories offer you no nutrition.

What's a Moderate Amount of Alcohol?

Alcohol should be consumed in moderation, and this applies to both people with diabetes and those without diabetes. For women, a moderate amount of alcohol is one serving per day and no more than 3 per day. For men, a moderate amount of alcohol is 2 servings per day and no more than 4 per day. Don't average this amount over a few days or drink it all in one or two days. Avoid binge drinking, which is technically defined as drinking four or more drinks for women and five or more drinks for men within a two-hour time frame.

What's a Serving of Alcohol?

Table 16.1 shows serving sizes for many of the types of alcoholic beverages people drink.

Get to Know Yourself

If you want to change your habits, you need to take stock of your current habits with drinking alcohol. Ask yourself these questions about your alcohol intake.

- How many times a day or a week do I drink alcohol and how much?
- What kinds of alcohol do I drink?

TABLE 16.1 Serving Sizes for Alcoholic Beverages	
Alcoholic beverage	**Serving size**
Beer	
–light (less than 4.5% abv)	12 fl oz
–regular (about 5% abv)	12 fl oz
–dark (more than 5.7% abv)	12 fl oz
Distilled spirits (80 or 60 proof):	
vodka, rum, gin, whiskey, tequila	1 1/2 fl oz
Liqueur (53 proof)	1 fl oz
Sake	1 fl oz
Wine	
–champagne/sparkling	5 fl oz
–dessert (sherry)	3 1/2 fl oz
–dry, red or white (10% abv)	5 fl oz

abv stands for "alcohol by volume." It is a measure of how much alcohol is contained in a beverage.

- Do I mix alcohol with a calorie-containing mixer (such as juice, regular soda, or tonic water) or a noncaloric mixer?

- How often would I like to include alcohol in my healthy eating plan?

The Upside and Downside of Alcohol

Upside

From a health standpoint, there are a few benefits of a moderate intake of alcohol spread out over several days a week. Regular intake of moderate amounts of alcohol over time can increase insulin sensitivity and decrease insulin resistance. This is due to alcohol's anti-inflammatory effect and is exactly the response you want to slow your prediabetes or type 2 diabetes. It results in lower fasting glucose; lower risk of heart disease, strokes, and death from all causes; and can improve thinking and memory. Indeed, a great list of health benefits!

When it comes to diabetes, moderate amounts of alcohol have little short- or long-term effects on blood glucose levels. But more than three drinks per day can, over time, make blood glucose control a challenge.

If you do not currently drink alcohol, don't start drinking alcohol due to its health benefits. There are many other, more powerful actions you can take to achieve your health goals, such as getting adequate sleep most nights, not smoking, and being physically active.

Downside

Alcohol slows down physical and mental reaction time and can impair good judgment, including making healthier food choices. The effects of alcohol are dangerous for anyone, diabetes or no diabetes, behind the wheel of a car or for people near an intoxicated driver.

Excess alcohol consumption can cause a host of health problems. Women who are thinking of becoming pregnant or are currently pregnant or breast-feeding should consult with their health-care provider about whether it's safe for them to consume alcohol.

From a nutrition standpoint, alcohol serves up calories with no nutrition. A couple of glasses of wine at dinner can quickly add up to 200 calories. If you are trying to eat 1,400–1,600 calories a day, 200 calories is nearly 15% of your calories. If you use up 200 calories as alcohol, you'll be hard pressed to eat all the nutrients you need and stay within your calorie limits.

If you have diabetes, depending on the blood glucose–lowering medications you take, alcohol can cause blood glucose to drop too low (hypoglycemia). Hypoglycemia can occur hours after you consume alcohol. Be sure to check with your health-care provider to verify if any of the medications you take may cause hypoglycemia. Some medications that can potentially cause hypoglycemia are listed in Table 16.2.

TABLE 16.2	Blood Glucose–Lowering Medications that May Cause Hypoglycemia*	
Category name	Generic name	Brand names in U.S.
Sulfonylureas	Glimepiride Glipizide Glyburide	Amaryl Glucotrol, Glucotrol XL Diabeta, Micronase, Glynase
D-Phenylalanine derivative	Nateglinide	Starlix
Meglintinide	Repaglinide	Prandin
Amylin analog	Pramlintide	Symlin
GLP-1 agonist	Exenatide	Byetta
Insulin	Lispro, aspart, glulisine, regular, glargine, detemir, NPH, degludec	Humalog, NovoLog, Apidra, Lantus, Levemir, Humulin, Novolin, Tresiba

*This is not a complete list of medications. Check with your health-care provider to see if any medications you may be taking can cause hypoglycemia. Be aware that combination pills may contain both a medication that can cause hypoglycemia and one that does not.

Fitting Alcohol into Your Eating Plan

Current guidelines from the American Diabetes Association suggest that you factor moderate amounts of alcohol into your eating plan in addition to the calories you consume from foods and calorie-containing non alcoholic beverages. If you want to lose weight, remember that the calories from alcohol can add up quickly.

What Kind of Alcohol Is Best?

Red or white wine, bourbon or whiskey, or regular or light beer? Though you may hear red wine is best, and some fans of the Mediterranean eating plan still promote red wine as best, research doesn't show that one type of alcohol offers more health benefits than another. No matter what type of alcohol you drink, it is best to drink as few calories and grams of carbohydrate from mixers as you can, so avoid mixed drinks with juice and grenadine syrup or ones with regular soda. For mixers, stick with club soda, sparkling mineral water, diet tonic water, water, diet soda, tomato or V8 juice, Bloody Mary mix, or coffee (for a hot drink).

Alcohol Adds Flavor, Not Fat

A bit of wine, sherry, or liqueur can enhance the taste of foods and adds just a few calories. Alcohol is a wonderful low-fat cooking ingredient. You might stock red and white cooking wine, sherry, and liqueurs (clear ones, not creamy) in your pantry. Here are just a few culinary ideas.

- Add sherry to a marinade for chicken or meat.
- Pour red cooking wine into a tomato sauce.
- Use white cooking wine in a poaching liquid.
- Add orange liqueur to a fruit salad.
- Dress up coffee with a spot of hazelnut liqueur.
- Drizzle a tablespoon of raspberry liqueur on frozen yogurt.
- Poach fruit in red wine.

Tips to Sip By

- Don't drink alcoholic beverages when your blood glucose is too low.

- If you take a medication that can cause low blood glucose (see Table 16.2), have a snack or meal with the alcohol if your blood glucose is too low when you start to drink.

- Check your blood glucose levels more often when you drink alcohol. These checks will help you learn more about the effect of alcohol on your body.

- Before you drive a vehicle after you have had a drink, check your blood glucose to make sure it is in a safe range. Do not drive if you believe you've had too much to drink or you risk going too low.

- The symptoms of intoxication and hypoglycemia can be similar. People may confuse these two and might not provide you with the proper treatment. Make sure you drink safely and wear a medical ID that says you have diabetes.

- Slowly sip a drink to make it last.

- Make a glass of wine last longer by making it a "spritzer." Mix the wine with sparkling water, club soda, or diet ginger ale.

- Choose light beer over regular beer if you like it and want to save a few calories.

- When you drink alcohol, have a no-calorie beverage, like water, club soda, or diet soda, on the side to quench your thirst.

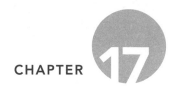

CHAPTER

Combination, Convenience, and Free Foods

What's Ahead?

➡ Definitions of combination and convenience foods and how to fit them in your healthy eating plan.

➡ Definition of free foods and how to fit them in your healthy eating plan.

➡ Serving sizes and nutrition numbers for combination, convenience, and free foods.

Combination Foods Defined

You've read a lot in section 2 about foods that fit nicely into the different food groups. The way these foods divide into food groups makes sense most of the time: apples in the fruit group, barley in the starch group, and pork chops in the protein group. That's all fine, but you likely also regularly enjoy combination foods or dishes: bean burritos, beef stew, Chinese stir-fry, or minestrone soup; the list is nearly endless. Take one example, bean burritos. Foods in this dish come from several food groups. Beans and tortillas are in the starch group, cheese is in the protein group, and lettuce, onion, and tomato are all in the vegetable group.

Convenience Foods Defined

Think of convenience foods as the packaged foods you buy in the supermarket or convenience store that are just one or a few steps away from being ready to eat. Frozen pizza, a box of macaroni and cheese, and a lean frozen entrée are all convenience foods. Over the years, convenience foods have become more and more popular with Americans.

If there's one benefit of convenience foods for people with diabetes, it's that they generally have Nutrition Facts labels and ingredients on the packaging. This can help you know what you're eating, but it is certainly not a reason to prefer convenience foods over less processed foods. Later in this chapter, you'll find tips to help you make healthier convenience-food choices.

Got a Recipe?

If you're going to prepare a favorite old recipe or try out a new one, learn how to fit a serving of a recipe into your healthy eating plan by following these steps:

1. Write down the amount of each ingredient used in the recipe. There are websites that provide tools for you to do this quicker and easier. Try www.myfitnesspal.com/recipe/calculator.

2. Find the grams of carbohydrate, protein, and fat in the amount of each ingredient. Use an online nutrient database resource such as the American Diabetes Association's My Food Advisor (http://tracker.diabetes.org) or the USDA's searchable food database (http://ndb.nal.usda.gov).

3. Divide the total grams of carbohydrate, protein, and fat by the number of portions you will serve from the recipe.

4. If you think you'll prepare the recipe again, record the nutrition information per servings on the recipe. Then you'll have it for the future.

Here's an example using a recipe for Vegetarian Mexican Chili.

VEGETARIAN MEXICAN CHILI

Ingredients	Amount	Carb (g)	Protein (g)	Fat (g)
Chopped onions	1 cup	16	2	0
Chopped red pepper	3/4 cup	7	1	0
Chopped green pepper	3/4 cup	5	1	0
Minced garlic	2 tsp	2	0	0
Kidney beans	2 (16-oz) cans	160	54	4
Stewed tomatoes	2 (14 1/2-oz) cans	55	8	2
Tomato paste	1 (6-oz) can	32	7	1
Bulgur, dry	2/3 cup	70	11	1
Chili powder	1 1/2 Tbsp	0	0	0
Cumin, ground	1 tsp	0	0	0
Totals for whole recipe		**347**	**84**	**8**
Totals for 1 portion (1/6 of recipe)		**58**	**14**	**1**

Think about the food groups represented in this recipe. You've got onions, peppers, and tomatoes from the vegetable group and beans and bulgur from the starch group. Spices and seasonings like garlic, chili powder, and cumin have essentially no calories, so they are free foods.

Subtract the amounts from the amounts in one portion of the recipe as shown in Table 17.1. Note that there are a few grams of carbohydrate, protein, and fat remaining, but this is close enough. When you calculate food group servings, the goal is to come as close as possible without going over the calculated nutrients. One portion of this Vegetarian Mexican Chili contains 3 starch and 2 vegetable servings—a mighty healthy dish.

TABLE 17.1 Translating the Nutrients to Food Group Servings			
	Carbohydrate (g)	Protein (g)	Fat (g)
Totals for 1 portion (6 portions per recipe)	58	14	1
3 starch servings	–45	–9	–0
After starch calculation	13	5	1
2 vegetable servings	–10	–4	–0
Remainder	3	1	1

Fitting in Combination, Convenience, and Prepared Foods

Use this process to fit combination, convenience, or prepared foods into your eating plan. Get the grams of carbohydrate, protein, and fat in a serving of foods from the Nutrition Facts label if it's available. From the ingredients list, learn which ingredients contribute the three calorie-containing nutrients. Use this information and the process above to figure out the servings from the different food groups.

Even better, some foods already include the food group servings to help you easily fit them into your eating plan.

Putting Together Meals with Convenience Foods

If you use some of the healthier convenience foods, you can quickly put together nutritious meals. For example, combine a frozen pizza with a salad that you make at home or buy, and then add an apple for dessert. You may choose a frozen entrée that is healthy and combine it with a serving of leftover broccoli, a slice of whole-wheat bread, and glass of fat-free milk. There are many convenience foods available. The following examples show you how to use them to your advantage to put together healthy meals.

SAMPLE MEAL PLAN **WITH CONVENIENCE FOODS**

BREAKFAST: Frozen Waffles

2 frozen whole-grain waffles	2 starch, 1 fat
1 1/4 cups sliced strawberries	1 fruit
1 cup fat-free milk	1 milk

LUNCH: Frozen Pizza

2 slices pizza topped with red peppers,	3 starch
tomatoes, and mushrooms	2 protein
	2 vegetable
	2 fat
1 cup fat-free, sugar-free strawberry yogurt	1 milk
1 small banana sliced into yogurt	1 fruit

DINNER: Frozen Entrée

Chinese Chicken Stir-Fry	2 starch
	1 vegetable
	3 protein
	2 fat
1 small whole-wheat dinner roll	1 starch
Salad with lettuce, cucumbers,	1 vegetable
carrots, and sliced tomato	
1 tsp extra-virgin olive oil	1 fat
2 Tbsp balsamic vinegar	free food
1 cup fat-free milk	1 milk

Choosing Healthier Convenience Foods

Convenience foods are not generally as healthy as if you make the item from scratch. Many packaged items and frozen foods are higher in sodium and contain unnecessary additives and preservatives. Some fresh fruits and vegetables that are pre-washed, cut up, and ready to eat are just as healthy but offer the convenience of several steps being done for you. Some packaged convenience foods may contain more fat and/or sodium. You need to read Nutrition Facts and ingredients before placing any convenience food in your shopping cart.

Sure, it would be best to make all your food from scratch, but most people don't have the time or inclination these days. Try to use as few convenience foods as you can, and select healthier convenience foods when you buy them. For example, choose lower-sodium options whenever they are available, such as soup, broth, or canned vegetables. Choose frozen vegetables that don't have special sauces or seasonings. Add your own herbs, spices, and seasonings. Remember that processed foods contribute about three-quarters of the sodium we eat.

Table 17.3 at the end of this chapter provides the serving sizes for some popular convenience and combination foods, along with their calorie, carbohydrate, protein, fat, saturated fat, and sodium content. Check them out.

Free Foods

Free foods, as defined by the American Diabetes Association, contain less than 20 calories or less than 5 grams of carbohydrate per serving. You'll find the list of free foods in Table 17.2 (also at the end of this chapter), along with serving size (if one is indicated). If a free food is listed with a serving size, it means that it contains more than a few calories and should be limited to no more than 3 servings a day. Spread servings of free foods like this throughout the day. If you eat all 3 servings at one time, this amount of the food might raise your blood glucose level. Foods listed without a serving size can be eaten whenever you want in whatever quantity (within reason) you want.

TABLE 17.2 Serving Sizes for Free Foods	
Food	**Serving Size**
LOW-CARBOHYDRATE FOODS	
Candy, hard (regular or sugar-free)	1 piece
Fruits	
Cranberries, sweetened with sugar substitute	1/2 cup
Rhubarb, sweetened with sugar substitute	1/2 cup
Gelatin dessert, sugar-free, any flavor	
Gum, sugar-free	
Jam or jelly, light or no-sugar-added	2 tsp
Salad greens (such as arugula, chicory, endive, escarole, leaf or iceberg lettuce, purslane, romaine, radicchio, spinach, watercress)	
Sugar substitutes (artificial sweeteners)	
Syrup, sugar-free	2 Tbsp
Vegetables: any *raw* nonstarchy vegetables (such as broccoli, cabbage, carrots, cucumber, tomato)	1/2 cup
Vegetables: any *cooked* nonstarchy vegetables (such as carrots, cauliflower, green beans)	1/4 cup
REDUCED-FAT OR FAT-FREE FOODS	
Cream cheese, fat-free	1 Tbsp (1/2 oz)
Coffee creamers, nondairy	
liquid, flavored	1 1/2 tsp
liquid, sugar-free, flavored	4 tsp
powdered, flavored	1 tsp
powdered, sugar-free, flavored	2 tsp
Margarine spread	
fat-free	1 Tbsp
reduced-fat	1 tsp
Mayonnaise	
fat-free	1 Tbsp
reduced-fat	1 tsp
Mayonnaise-style salad dressing	
fat-free	1 Tbsp
reduced-fat	2 tsp
Salad dressing	
fat-free	1 Tbsp
fat-free, Italian	2 Tbsp

continued

TABLE 17.2 *continued*	
Food	**Serving Size**
Sour cream, fat-free or reduced-fat	1 Tbsp
Whipped topping	
light or fat-free	2 Tbsp
regular	1 Tbsp
CONDIMENTS	
Barbecue sauce	2 tsp
Ketchup	1 Tbsp
Chili sauce, sweet, tomato-type	2 tsp
Horseradish	
Hot pepper sauce	
Lemon juice	
Miso	1 1/2 tsp
Mustard	
Honey	1 Tbsp
Yellow, Dijon, brown, horseradish-flavored, or wasabi-flavored	
Parmesan cheese, grated	1 Tbsp
Pickle relish (dill or sweet)	1 Tbsp
Pickles	
dill	1 1/2 medium
sweet, bread-and-butter	2 slices
sweet, gherkin	3/4 oz
Pimento	
Salsa	1/4 cup
Soy sauce, light or regular	1 Tbsp
Sweet-and-sour sauce	2 tsp
Taco sauce	1 Tbsp
Vinegar	
Worcestershire sauce	
Yogurt, any type	2 Tbsp
DRINKS/MIXES	
Bouillon, broth, consommé	
Bouillon or broth, low-sodium	
Carbonated or mineral water	
Club soda	
Cocoa powder, unsweetened	1 Tbsp
Coffee, unsweetened or with sugar substitute	
Diet soft drinks, sugar-free	

continued

TABLE 17.2 *continued*	
Food	**Serving Size**
Drink mixes (powder or liquid drops), sugar-free	
Tea, unsweetened or with sugar substitute	
Tonic water, sugar-free	
Water	
Water, flavored, sugar-free	
SEASONINGS	
Flavoring extracts (for example, vanilla, almond, peppermint)	
Garlic, fresh or powder	
Herbs, fresh or dried	
Kelp	
Nonstick cooking spray	
Spices	
Wine, used in cooking	

Source: Adapted from *Choose Your Foods: Food Lists for Diabetes.* Academy of Nutrition and Dietetics and American Diabetes Association, 2014.

TABLE 17.3	Serving Sizes, Calories, and Nutrients for Combination and Convenience Foods

Food	Serving Size
COMBINATION FOODS: ENTRÉES	
Chili with beans	1 cup
Lasagna with meat and sauce	1 cup
Macaroni and cheese	1 cup
Spaghetti, sauce, meatballs	1 cup
Stew, meat and vegetables	1 cup
Tuna noodle casserole	1 cup
Tuna or chicken salad	1/2 cup
COMBINATION FOODS: FROZEN ENTRÉES/MEALS	
Burrito (beef and bean)	1 burrito
Dinner-type meal, frozen	1 meal (16 oz)
Entrée or meal (<340 calories)	1 container (~9.5 oz)
Pizza, cheese, thin crust, frozen	1 1/4th of 12"
Pizza, meat topping, thin crust, frozen	1 1/4th of 12"
Pocket sandwich	1 sandwich
Pot pie, double crust	1 pie (7 oz)
COMBINATION FOODS: SALADS (DELI-STYLE)	
Coleslaw, deli-style	1/2 cup
Macaroni or pasta salad, deli-style	1/2 cup
Potato salad, mustard-type, deli-style	1/2 cup
COMBINATION FOODS: SOUPS	
Asian noodle soup (ramen-type)	1 cup
Chowder, made with milk	1 cup
Miso soup	1 cup
Rice soup (congee)	1 cup
Soup, bean	1 cup
Soup, chicken noodle, made with water	1 cup
Soup, cream of celery, made with water	1 cup
Soup, cream of mushroom, made with water	1 cup

Calories	Carb (g)	Protein (g)	Fat (g)	Saturated Fat (g)	Sodium (mg)
336	28.0	19.4	16.2	7.4	1,152
293	27.9	19.7	11.4	5.0	776
283	35.4	10.8	11.0	6.2	1,343
273	28.3	10.6	13.0	5.0	1,035
160	17.0	12.5	5.2	2.2	990
295	32.3	21.3	8.4	2.3	448
182	7.0	15.3	10.3	1.7	328
350	45.0	12.5	13.4	5.0	560
513	54.0	26.8	20.9	6.8	1,403
299	40.4	18.3	6.7	2.2	535
291	33.0	13.5	12.5	6.0	565
365	34.0	16.0	18.5	8.0	816
310	46.5	11.5	9.5	5.3	725
390	39.3	9.7	21.3	6.7	778
130	16.0	1.0	7.0	1.0	160
280	28.0	4.0	14.0	2.0	430
180	25.0	2.0	6.0	1.0	690
240	30.0	6.0	10.5	6.0	1,031
190	19.0	6.5	9.8	2.5	865
84	8.0	6.0	3.4	0.6	989
72	13.5	1.7	1.4	0.4	487
116	19.8	5.6	1.5	0.0	1,198
75	9.4	4.0	2.5	1.0	1,106
90	8.8	1.7	5.6	1.0	949
129	9.3	2.3	9.0	2.0	881

continued

TABLE 17.3 *continued*

Food	Serving Size
Soup, instant, 6 oz, prepared	1 envelope
Soup, instant, bean or lentil, prepared	1 container (2 oz)
Soup, split pea, made with water	1 cup
Soup, tomato, made with water	1 cup
Soup, vegetable beef, made with water	1 cup

Calories	Carb (g)	Protein (g)	Fat (g)	Saturated Fat (g)	Sodium (mg)
65	11.1	1.9	1.6	0.5	561
215	39.4	12.2	1.5	0.0	523
190	28.0	10.4	4.4	2.0	1,012
85	16.6	2.0	1.9	0.0	695
78	10.2	5.6	1.9	1.0	791

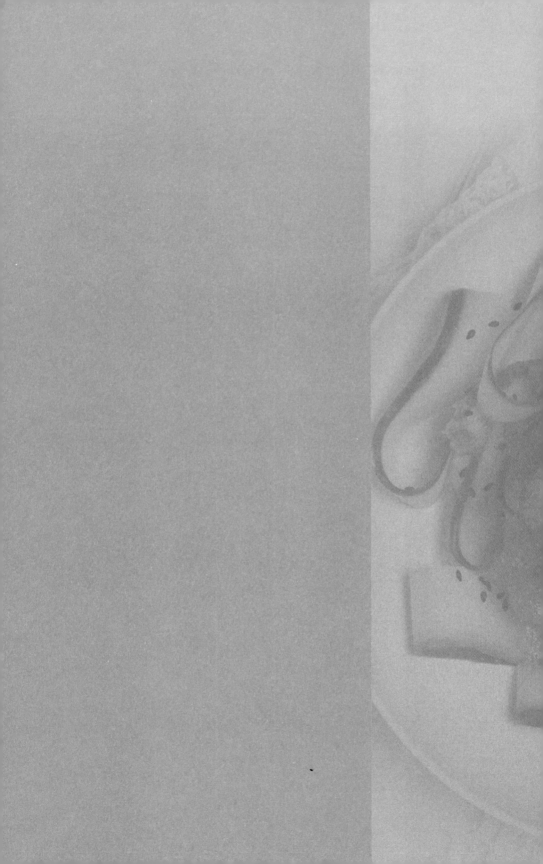

Put Healthy Eating for Diabetes Control into Action

CHAPTER 18

Change Your Food Choices and Eating Behaviors Slowly

What's Ahead?

→ How to set yourself up for success and deal positively with the challenges you'll face.

→ How to slowly make changes in the foods you choose in the supermarket, at restaurants, and other food venues.

→ Basics on how to adjust your eating habits to fit into your healthy lifestyle.

→ How to form a physical activity plan that fits your lifestyle.

→ How to identify what food choices and eating behaviors to change first, second, and over time.

→ How to define SMART behavior-change goals and set them.

→ How to track and evaluate your behavior-change efforts and build momentum for change.

Give Credit to Yourself Where and When It's Due

As you start to take stock of your current habits (yes, that's step one in this process) and you're doing the hard work to change them, give yourself lots of pats on the back for taking these positive steps. Pat yourself on the back for every little success you experience.

Here's what not to do. Don't beat yourself up if you don't succeed immediately. Changing your eating habits and food choices is hard work. It requires effort, fortitude, tenacity, and time. These changes don't happen overnight. Give yourself lots of "atta boy" or "atta girl" messages. Don't depend on others to do this. And don't expect perfection or the impossible. Remember, to err is human! You will have days when you're successful and days that just don't go as planned. At times life happens and gets in the way of your best intentions. Making real and long-lasting changes takes months or years to integrate into your new way of eating and living. You can get there!

Learn from both your positive and negative experiences. Figure out how to set yourself up for success and remove the self-imposed, as well as societal, hurdles and roadblocks. Don't let other people in your life—your family, health-care providers, or coworkers—expect too much of you, sabotage your efforts, or set you up for failure. All you can do and expect of yourself is the best you can do each day. Take one day at a time.

The good news is that making just a few small changes to eat healthier, reduce sedentary behavior (sitting), and be more physically active can have a huge effect on your weight, your body, how you feel, and your ABCs (blood glucose, blood pressure, and blood lipids).

When YOU are Ready, Willing, and Able to Change

People around you may tell you that you weigh too much or your blood glucose is out of control, but what do YOU think? Do YOU deny or accept that these are problems? If you deny that they're problems, you're not likely to be ready to set goals, or you may do it just to please others in your life. As long as you are in denial about your diabetes and the need to make lifestyle changes, your efforts aren't likely to succeed. You're likely to resent or be angry with the people who are pushing you to make changes.

To be successful at changing your behaviors, YOU need to acknowledge that YOU have a problem, and then YOU need to be ready, willing, and able to choose the changes to make. Experts in the science of human behavior change call this "readiness to change." People are typically at different points of their readiness to change for different behaviors. For example, you may be ready to increase your physical activity but don't want to hear about changing your eating habits or quitting smoking.

Experts in behavior change have shown that to start the process of making a behavior change, you need to accept that the behavior you want to change is a behavior that you believe you need to change. This is referred to as "importance"—changing the identified behavior has to be important to you. In essence, you have more reasons to change the behavior than to continue doing it as you have been.

You also must have confidence in your ability to change the behavior. Give these factors some thought when you choose behaviors you want to change: the importance to you and your confidence that you are able to make that change.

Take the slow and steady approach. Don't overestimate how many behaviors you can change and how fast you can change them. Experts say that you are more likely to succeed if you break the behaviors you are ready to change into small, easier-to-accomplish actions. Think of this as stringing together lots of tiny behavior changes. Over time and cumulatively, changing all of these behaviors will make a big difference.

Choosing What to Change First

You won't be able to choose which behavior to change first unless you get to know yourself and your habits better. Be honest. Learn what, where, when, and how much you eat during the day, at night, on the weekends. Think about where and when you buy food. To start, keep a food diary for a few days (or longer if you can) to get a true picture of your food and eating habits. (See the form on page x in the Introduction, or use one of the many free online tracking tools or apps available today. Check out a few, and find one that works for you.) From your answers, you will see your strengths and areas where you could benefit from some changes. To help gain insight into your current food choices and eating habits, answer the "Get to Know Yourself" questions in each chapter in section 2.

Start by choosing one to three behavior changes that are important to you and you are confident are easy for you to tackle and succeed at changing. Make sure they offer you a big bang for your effort. Don't touch behaviors you don't feel ready, willing, or able to change—leave them for later.

If it feels right to you, select one eating-related change and another related to physical activity. If you successfully change one habit, you're more likely to tackle the next more eagerly. For example, an easy change for you might be to eat healthier food for your nighttime snacks or to switch from whole milk to fat-free milk. A more difficult change would be to start eating breakfast if you never do.

When you set behavior-change goals, it's important to make them realistic. If your goals are too general or overly ambitious, you won't achieve them. Set SMART goals. Each letter of the word SMART is an element of a realistic behavior change goal (Table 18.1).

TABLE 18.1 SMART Goals

Letter	Abbreviation	Definition
S	Specific	Narrowly define your goal.
M	Measurable	Choose a frequency for the goal. How many times a day or week will you do this?
A	Attainable	Make the goal challenging but something that you can accomplish.
R	Realistic	Make the goal something you can do within the confines of your current life.
T	Time-frame specific	Limited in time frame—set short-term goals which are easier to achieve.

Examples of SMART Behavior-Change Goals

Current Behavior #1: You eat breakfast on the run from a fast-food spot or the cafeteria at work, Monday through Friday. Your usual choices are a sausage biscuit, a bagel with a thick layer of regular cream cheese, or a huge muffin and a banana.

Behavior-Change Goal: For the next month (short time frame), on 2 days each week (measurable), I will choose one of these healthier breakfasts: a whole-wheat English muffin with jelly and a small banana, or a half bagel with light or fat-free cream cheese with an orange or half grapefruit (specific and realistic).

Current Behavior #2: You realize that you consume little or no milk or yogurt over the course of a week.

Behavior-Change Goal: For the next 2 weeks (short time frame), on 3 days each week (measurable), I will drink an 8-ounce carton of fat-free milk with my lunch or take a container of refrigerated fat-free, sugar-free fruited yogurt to eat as an afternoon snack (specific and realistic).

Set at least one and not more than three behavior-change goals at a time. Record your goals on your smartphone, a tablet, an online program, or simply a pad of paper. Use whatever tool works best for you. Keep your goals in a convenient location, where you will see them often. Print them out and post them on the refrigerator, bathroom mirror, or bedroom mirror, or keep them close in your purse or wallet.

Now, it's your turn. Write down a few goals based on what you've learned about your eating habits.

Track Your Goals and Actions

People don't generally like to keep records, whether it's food choices, physical activity, blood glucose, or weight. It's time consuming and a bother. But, and this is a big but, studies continually show that regular record keeping is one of the most important factors in helping you make and maintain behavior changes to accomplish your goals, from losing weight and keeping it off to improving your diabetes care. It's all about accountability to yourself.

It's valuable for you to keep records of your blood glucose checks, the foods and amounts you eat, the physical activity you do, and whatever else you and your providers believe will help you achieve your goals. But take it slow. Choose easy targets for record keeping. Then over time add new subjects to your records. You may want to keep records about one aspect of your process for behavior change for a period of time and then change to tracking something else. Again, try different approaches, and zero in on what works best for you.

Keep records in whatever way is best and most efficient for you. Pen and paper is fine. However, you may want to investigate online tools or apps that might make the job easier. Online resources, devices, and apps are constantly evolving. New ones are available on a near-daily basis, and many are free. Read descriptions and reviews of online tools and apps to find the resources that are best for you. Remember that there's nothing magical about these online tools. They only assist you if you use them regularly and over time.

To get and keep you going initially, make sure you experience success with an easy-to-change behavior. Keep on practicing this one behavior. Next identify a few more tiny behaviors you can successfully change. Over time you'll see that success breeds success. Plus, making these incremental behavior changes will become easier.

Evaluate Your Success

The last lap in every behavior change cycle is to evaluate your success. Use your records to see whether you successfully made the behavior changes you set for yourself or if you need to revise your goals. The records you have kept can help you identify your stumbling blocks, actions that you find helpful, and the effects of tweaks in your diabetes regimen.

Some Nutrition, Weight Control, and Physical Activity Online Tools

- My Fitness Pal (www.myfitnesspal.com).
- FitDay (www.fitday.com).
- SparkPeople (www.sparkpeople.com).
- My Food Diary (www.myfoodiary.com).
- Calorie King (www.calorieking.com).
- Super Tracker (www.supertracker.usda.gov).
- Weight Watchers (www.weightwatchers.com).

Some Diabetes-Focused Tools

- mysugr (mysugr.com).
- American Diabetes Association My Food Advisor (http://tracker.diabetes.org).
- Glucose Buddy (www.glucosebuddy.com).
- Diabetes In Check (this is a mobile app).
- Diabetic Connect (www.diabeticconnect.com).
- Diabetes App (this is a mobile app).
- dbees (dbees.com).

As you evaluate your success, ask yourself these questions:

- Did I meet my goals?
- If not, why not?
- Were they unrealistic?
- Was the time frame too long?

If you were successful, give yourself a BIG pat (or two) on the back and a non food reward. Take the time to think about what worked for you and what helped you succeed. Apply what you learned to your future goals. If you didn't reach your goals, then make your goals easier to accomplish, or choose another goal that you can achieve more easily.

Your Next Step

Start the behavior-change cycle again. Choose a few new goals to work on. Set them using the SMART goals format.

Practicing a new behavior for 2 weeks or a month does not mean that this new behavior has become a lifelong behavior. It's easy to slip back into old behaviors. They're familiar and you've practiced them a long time. Practice the new behaviors faithfully over time. Research shows that it takes at least 6 months before the new behaviors become your way of life. For instance, now you always remember to stick a piece of fruit in your briefcase before you leave home in the morning and eat it during the afternoon. Maybe you automatically choose a garden salad with light dressing at a fast-food restaurant rather than french fries, or you make sure to get your 20-minute after-lunch walk at least 3 days a week because you know you'll feel sluggish in the afternoon otherwise.

Keep in mind that stressful (positive or negative) life events or schedule disruptions may get you off your new healthy reflexes. Be on the lookout for these events. If you see your new behaviors slowly going by the wayside, quickly go back to the successful strategies you implemented to make your changes.

If you put this behavior-change process into action, before long you'll find yourself at a healthier weight. You may also find that your ABCs improve. Always keep in mind that you may need to start, increase, or add a blood glucose–lowering medication to achieve your ABCs. Don't resist this effort by your providers to keep you healthy. Regardless of the medications you have to take to hit your ABC goals, healthy eating and physical activity always assist your efforts!

Create a Positive Partnership with Your Provider

Your health-care providers play an important role in supporting your healthy behavior changes. Here are tips for working with your providers to make the most out of your appointments.

- Get organized for your visit. Bring any important health records with you. Think about and write down the most important things you'd like to discuss or questions you have, and use them as a checklist for your appointment.

- Ask what your target ABC levels should be, if you don't know.

- Ask what your before and after eating blood glucose levels should be. This can help you identify any changes you need to make in your lifestyle and medication routines.

- Talk about any blood glucose patterns you're observing, and have your results ready to share. For example, you may find that it's always higher after dinner than after lunch, or maybe you regularly experience a low blood glucose reading after breakfast.

- Be honest with your providers about your current lifestyle and what you are ready, willing, and able to change. Work in partnership with your provider to create a diabetes care plan that works for you. This can enable you and your provider to dance together rather than feel like you're in a wrestling match.

- Ask for help if you need it. Ask about any programs or specialists that may be available to support your efforts.

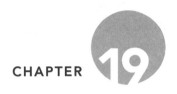

Planning: A BIG Key to Healthy Eating

What's Ahead?

→ Why planning, from foods and meals to market to table, is your key to healthier eating.

→ How to stock your pantry and refrigerator for healthy eating.

→ Steps to take before you leave for the supermarket.

→ How to pick quick and easy family-favorite recipes and have foods for a few on hand.

→ Tips to shop smart in the supermarket aisles.

Planning Is Your Key to Healthier Eating

To eat healthfully day to day and week to week, you need to get into a groove. Getting into that groove requires regular planning. This chapter gives you the tools to integrate planning into your regular routine. First, spend a few minutes to plan the meals you'll prepare and eat during the next week, and think about the other foods you need and want to have accessible. Now, draft your shopping list. Assess the foods you have on hand and those you'll need to buy. These steps may seem time-consuming, but the shopping trap that many people fall into costs you in three ways: health, time, and money. Here's why:

Health

When you don't plan, you're more likely to make food decisions when you are hungry, tired, and vulnerable to unhealthy choices. You're more likely to fall back on convenience items and restaurant meals. If you eat this way, it's likely you'll end up eating fewer fruits, vegetables, and whole grains and more high-fat meat, fat, sugars, and sodium. Conversely, when you do the all-important planning, healthy choices are easier to make. Keep those unhealthy foods out of the house as much as possible. Replace them with healthier grab-and-go options.

Time

If you wait to think about what you'll make for dinner until your ride home from work or other daily activities, you're more likely to select convenience or restaurant foods. Now, if you have foods ready at home for quick dinners, you can have a healthy meal on the table in no time. These healthy meals don't need to be fancy. Consider a slice or two of frozen pizza topped with vegetables alongside a quick salad, a shrimp or chicken stir-fry served on top of brown rice or quinoa that you've made several servings of in advance, or a serving of leftovers you defrosted that morning with a serving of a starch and frozen vegetables.

Money

It is far more cost-effective to prepare meals at home. If you're buying your foods at convenience stores, ordering takeout, having food delivered, eating at restaurants, or cruising through the drive-thru, you'll be spending more money on less food and likely less healthy food than you would be if you were cooking at home.

Carve Out Planning Time

Carve out time to plan your meals; take stock of your pantry, refrigerator, and freezer; and develop your concise and complete weekly shopping list. Once you make planning a consistent activity in your life, it will become habit. You'll be able to do your planning in no more than 15 minutes. It may take a bit more time if you are feeding a household.

To start integrating the habit of planning into your life, figure out a convenient time to do it. Perhaps what's best for you is early in the morning or late at night while winding down, or on a Sunday morning before your weekly supermarket run. Mark this planning period on your calendar so it becomes a regular part of your routine.

More and more services are popping up online that make meal planning, shopping, and food preparation easier. The pros and cons of these popular services are listed in Table 19.1.

Plan Your Meals

Decide what foods you'll eat and what meals you'll prepare for the week. Need a few new meal ideas? Seek out healthy recipes from myriad resources: read magazines like **Diabetes Forecast** or other diabetes- or health-oriented publications, go online to healthy recipe websites, or grab a cookbook or two from your shelf to search for inspiration. But don't challenge yourself too much. Be realistic about what you'll have time to prepare. Think about your schedule to determine if you will eat every meal at home or if some days you'll be eating restaurant meals. Consider if you need to make any meals ahead of time or if you will prepare meals on the spot.

Think about the goals you set in chapter 18. If one of your goals is to eat more fruit, think about when you'll eat it and which fruits

TABLE 19.1	Pros and Cons of Meal-Planning and Delivery Services	
Service	Pros & cons	Sample services
Shopping Place your grocery order online. Have foods delivered to your door.	**Pros:** Save time and reduce impulse purchases. **Cons:** Delivery fees for some companies.	• Availability varies by location. • National options include Amazon, Walmart, Netgrocer, Vitacost, EthnicGrocer.
Meal planning Use an online service to customize menu plans, get recipes, and generate shopping lists.	**Pros:** Takes the grunt work out of planning. All you need to do is shop, cook, and eat. **Cons:** Most have a monthly fee.	• Relish, Fresh20, eMeals, Saving Dinner, Six O'Clock Scramble, Plan to Eat.
Meal delivery You choose the meals; then they're delivered fresh, frozen, or raw, depending on the service.	**Pros:** All or most of the work is done for you. **Cons:** Often expensive and not all services meet special dietary needs, like those of people with diabetes.	• Availability varies by location. • Options include Plated, Blue Apron, BistroMD, Seattle Sutton, Hello Fresh, The Purple Carrot.

you'll need to have. If your goal is to eat 2 servings of fruit a day, perhaps try to eat one at breakfast and then bring the second one in your brown-bag lunch. Your meal planning and shopping list should always incorporate your behavior-change goals.

Which Foods Do You Need?

Once you know the foods you'll want to make, take an inventory of what you currently have. Check your grocery list for items that you may already have in the freezer, refrigerator, and pantry. A helpful tactic is to keep a running inventory list of all of the foods you have in your house, so you can immediately make notes when you run low on or out of something. Doing this will save you extra trips to the grocery store and help you save money. Also, if you have the

Tips to Plan Meals and Menus

- Choose quick-to-fix recipes. They can save you during busy, time-crunched days.
- Get to know and make use of some of the ready-to-eat foods in the supermarket. They can make preparing meals at home easier.
- Try to incorporate leftovers into your plan, so you can cook once and eat twice.
- Make a double batch of a recipe and then freeze half for another week.
- Develop a list of 5–10 of your family's favorite easy recipes. Always have the ingredients on hand for 3–5 of these recipes. Easy, quick-to-fix recipes share certain common features.
    - Have no more than 5–8 ingredients.
    - Include easy-to-find ingredients.
    - Are simple to prepare.
    - Follow healthy eating guidelines.
    - Pair well with or contain vegetables and whole grains.
    - Please everyone in the family.
    - Leftovers store well.
    - Travel well as a brown-bag lunch.

space, keep a backup supply of some staples, such as salad dressings, oil, canned broth, and frozen pizza.

Create a Shopping List

Spend a few minutes at your computer to create your personal food inventory, or use one of the many online resources to do this. This inventory will also double as your household shopping list. Here's how you create one.

Think about the foods you usually buy and always want to have in your pantry. Put these into your food inventory. Divide the foods you buy into categories based on the floorplan of your usual super-market. Obviously, you buy non food items in the supermarket as well. Put them on your list, too. Take the list and look in your freezer, refrigerator, and pantry to make sure you haven't missed putting anything on your inventory. Add these in. If you want to keep a certain number on hand or make note of the size that you buy, record this information. When you check your house before going shopping, use your food inventory to make sure you're stocked at the levels you want. Now you have an inventory of the foods your household uses and likes to keep on hand.

If you've created your food inventory on a computer, print out a few copies. Always keep a few food inventory lists sight in your kitchen, like on a bulletin board. Update your food inventory as the foods you want in the house change.

Your food inventory also doubles as your grocery shopping list. Take your list to the supermarket with you, and let it guide your purchases.

This simple tool can greatly speed your planning as well as your shopping trips. It can also limit what you drop in your cart. It may take some time to put these planning steps into action, but they will save you time and money and help you eat healthier.

Get Ready to Shop

You've planned your meals and snacks, taken your food inventory, and are ready to shop. Now, with your food inventory in hand, you're ready for your organized, time-efficient trip to the supermar-ket. Few people relish this trip. Supermarkets keep getting larger. There are endless aisles, food and nutrition labels to read, and ever-lengthening ingredients lists. Use these tactics to make the most of your trips to the market and to save you time and money:

- **Shop at the same supermarket.** Because you know where things are, you'll shop faster. Ask for help to locate an item as soon as you need it. Generally, the employees can save you time and energy looking for items.

Sample Food Inventory

Dairy	Fresh Fruit	Fresh Vegetables	Breads and Starches	Cereals	Frozen Foods
Fat-free milk, 1/2 gallon	Apples (4)	Lettuce, bag	Whole-wheat sandwich	Cheerios	Pizza, cheese (2)
Yogurt, plain, quart	Bananas (3)	Lettuce, other	Raisin	Granola	Peas
Yogurt, fruit, 6 ounce (5)	Grapefruit	Peppers, red and green	Tortillas	Bran Flakes	Corn
Cottage cheese, 1%	Oranges (6)	Mushrooms	Pita pockets	Shredded Wheat	Fruit
Parmesan cheese	Mango	Red onion	Rice, brown	Oat bran	
Jarlsberg cheese	Blue-berries	Onions	Couscous	Oatmeal	
Eggs	Kiwi	Potatoes	Pasta, whole-wheat		
Margarine, stick	Other	Cucumber	Grains (quinoa, barley, millet)		
Margarine, tub		Carrots			
Orange juice with calcium, 1/2 gallon		Tomatoes, grape			
Other		Tomatoes, whole			
		Vegetables for week			

- **Shop as infrequently as you can.** Your shopping frequency depends on your family's size, the amount of fresh produce you buy, how much you can carry, and so on. The more organized you are and the more storage space you have, the less frequently you need to shop.

- **Go to the supermarket when it is not crowded.** Many supermarkets are open 24 hours a day. Try to avoid shopping between 5 and 7 P.M. That's typically the dinnertime rush.

- **Shop at one store where you can buy almost everything.** Limit stopping here for this and going there for that.

- **Avoid shopping when you are hungry.** An empty stomach means a fuller shopping cart.

- **Let your food inventory be your guide.** Try not to throw in impulse items. (It may be best to leave the kids at home if you can.)

- **Remember, the healthiest foods are often around the perimeter of the supermarket.** Fruits and vegetables are along one wall, meats and poultry down another, and dairy foods along another wall.

- **Do not walk every aisle.** If you know you do not need items on a particular aisle, move on to the next, especially if there are aisles with foods you are better off leaving behind.

- **Read Nutrition Facts labels and ingredients lists to make sure you know what you're buying and that the food fits into your meal plan.** Review the helpful information in chapter 21 in the "Guides for the Supermarket Aisles" section.

- **Find and buy the same foods week after week that satisfy your taste buds and nutrition needs.** If you do this, then you don't spend too much time reading food labels. Watch for bargains and new foods. Variety is good, so long as it meets your eating goals.

CHAPTER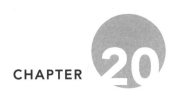

Control Your Portions

What's Ahead?

- → How portion sizes have grown.
- → Tools and tactics to tackle portion control.
- → Strategies to control portions in your kitchen and dining room.
- → Strategies and tools to control portions when you eat restaurant foods and meals.

Portion Distortion

Portions of foods, whether you eat them at home or in restaurants, are often oversized. Research shows that people will eat more if they serve themselves or have large dishes put in front of them. This is even true for young children.

Portions began to grow about 20–30 years ago, and so did the number of people who became overweight and obese. Portions are not the only reason people have gained weight, but they're one BIG factor. To gain some perspective on how much portions have grown, consider the comparisons in Table 20.1 from the Portion Distortion Quiz from the National Heart, Lung, and Blood Institute (www. nhlbi.nih.gov).

People have lost sight of reasonable food portions! Have you? To control calories and lose weight, it's critical to reacquaint yourself with reasonable portion sizes. First, learn the servings of food you need to eat by checking the serving sizes of the foods provided at the end of each chapter in section 2.

Calories Here and There Add Up

Losing weight and keeping it off are difficult tasks. Accomplishing these goals can come down to avoiding a few hundred extra calories above your daily target day after day. It may not seem possible that an extra half cup of carrots, a teaspoon of a healthy oil, or a tablespoon of mayonnaise makes a big difference, but those calories add up. Avoiding extra calories here and there is complicated by the fact that people often underestimate the amount of food and calories they eat. Some research estimates this total is about 500

TABLE 20.1	Portion Sizes: 20 Years Ago versus Today	
Food	20 Years Ago	Today
Bagel	3" diameter, 140 calories	6" diameter, 350 calories
Cheeseburger	330 calories	590 calories
Spaghetti and meatballs	1 cup pasta, 3 small meatballs, 500 calories	2 cups pasta, 3 large meatballs, 1,000 calories
French fries	2 1/2 oz, 210 calories (today's small order at a fast-food restaurant)	7 oz, 610 calories (today's large order at a fast-food restaurant)
Turkey sandwich	1 sandwich on 2 slices of bread, 320 calories	1 sandwich on a large roll, 820 calories

calories a day. Conversely, people overestimate the amount of physical activity they do and the calories it burns.

You may overeat by 200, 300, or 400 calories each day. Maybe it's just a piece of fresh fruit that is larger than the serving size, an extra 1/3 cup of pasta, or an extra ounce of chicken. You might think it's okay because these foods are on your "healthy" eating plan, but these extra calories can add up to enough calories to make a difference in your weight loss and blood glucose management.

Portion-Control Tools

Here is a list of the portion-control tools you'll want to have handy in your kitchen. You probably already have them; however, they may need dusting off and more frequent use. Keeping them in view increases their use.

- Set of measuring spoons that includes 1/2 teaspoon, 1 teaspoon, 1/2 tablespoon, and 1 tablespoon. Don't try to measure with your silverware. Those spoons vary in size based on style and won't give you exact measurements.

- One-cup liquid measuring cup (glass or plastic) with lines showing measures for 1/4, 1/3, 1/2, 2/3, and 3/4 cup. To measure liquids correctly, set the cup down and bend down at eye level to make sure the liquid reaches the proper line.

- Set of dry-ingredient measuring cups that includes measures for 1/4 cup, 1/3 cup, 1/2 cup, and 1 cup. Choose the correct size for your serving, fill it to the top, and level it with the flat edge of a knife.

- Inexpensive ($5–$15) food scale to weigh foods measured in ounces, such as fresh fruit, bagels, potatoes, snack foods, cereals, baked goods, meats, fish, and cheese. More expensive food scales ($25–$200) are available. They measure more precisely in ounces, pounds, grams, or kilograms and may provide the gram weight and grams of carbohydrate based on an internal database, which can help with carb counting.

Using Your Measuring Tools Away from Home

It is one thing to have measuring equipment at home, but like most Americans, you probably eat many meals away from home. Have no fear! When you're on the road, your eyes and hands can become your portion-control tools. They work well at home, too, once you have the correct portions nailed down.

Don't underestimate a well-trained set of eyes. Your eyes are an invaluable measuring tool because they travel with you. Just make sure you keep them honest!

- Thumb tip (from tip of thumb to first knuckle) = 1 teaspoon.

- Thumb (from tip of thumb to second knuckle) = 1 tablespoon.

- Two fingers lengthwise = 1 ounce.

- Palm of hand = 3 ounces (a regular-size deck of cards is 3 ounces).

- Tight fist = 1/2 cup.

- Loose fist or cupped hand = 1 cup.

Note: These guidelines hold true for most women's hands, but some men's hands are much larger.

Check out the size of your hands in relation to various portions when you measure at home.

The Nutrition Facts Label on Food Packaging

The Nutrition Facts label is required on most packaged foods, and it is one of your best resources for portion control because the label must list the serving size. The FDA regulates the serving sizes on food labels. These are the serving sizes that food manufacturers must use to comply with the food-labeling law. They aren't necessarily the same serving sizes as the servings used in this book. The servings in this book are based on those in **Choose Your Foods: Food Lists for Diabetes,** a booklet published by the American Diabetes Association and the Academy of Nutrition and Dietetics.

Don't confuse the weight in grams listed next to the serving size with the grams of carbohydrate in one serving listed next to "Total Carbohydrate." They are different. All the nutrition information on the Nutrition Facts label is based on one serving. Use the serving sizes to help you learn what reasonable portions are. (The Nutrition Facts label is covered in the next chapter.)

From Raw to Cooked

How do you figure out how much cooked meat you get from raw meat, poultry, or seafood? Here are some guidelines:

* Raw meat with no bone: use 4 ounces raw to get 3 ounces cooked.

* Raw meat with bone: use 5 ounces raw to get 3 ounces cooked.

* Raw poultry with skin and bone: use 4 1/4–4 1/2 ounces to get 3 ounces cooked. The extra 1/4–1/2 ounce accounts for the skin. (Remove the skin before or after cooking.)

These guidelines may vary based on several factors: the cut of the meat, the amount of fat on the raw item and left on the cooked item, whether the cut contains bones or skin (for poultry), the cooking method you use (e.g., grilled, braised), and the degree of doneness to which you cook it (or it is cooked).

Weigh and Measure Foods Often

It's critical to familiarize yourself with reasonable portion sizes. The more you weigh and measure your foods and beverages, the more precise your portions will be. This will translate to success with controlling your weight and blood glucose levels. However, it's unrealistic to weigh and measure every food you eat every time you eat it, so here's a more realistic plan.

When you start to follow a healthy eating plan, weigh and measure your foods as frequently as possible. Take the time to get your portions in line with the amounts you should eat. Gradually, slack off a bit. Weigh and measure your foods less frequently. If you think you're estimating your portions accurately, weigh and measure your foods once a week, perhaps over the weekend, when you have a bit more time, or on Monday, the start of a new week. You may find that you serve yourself accurate portions of some foods, but you continue to overestimate others, like nuts, pasta, or meat.

Always weigh or measure new foods. Occasionally weigh or measure the foods and beverages you regularly eat to check that your portions are still accurate. Quiz yourself occasionally. Serve yourself dry cereal, a serving of cooked pasta or rice, or 3 ounces of cooked meat. Then use your tools to see how close you are to the actual portion size.

Go back to weighing and measuring your foods if you see your blood glucose levels change, your weight starts to level off or gradually climb, or if you are trying to maintain a certain weight or stop regaining weight you've lost.

Tips and Tricks to Control Portions at Home

- Use measuring tools to keep your eyes in line with proper portions. Always keep your measuring equipment (spoons, cups, and scale) in an easy-to-grab location. If you weigh and measure foods at home, you will have an easier time guesstimating portions when you eat out.

- Use smaller plates and bowls. Less food looks like more food on smaller plates. Dinner plates have gotten bigger and bigger. If you have a medium-size plate, use that for dinner. You'll avoid overfilling your plate.

- Don't serve family style. Avoid putting bowls, pots, or casserole pans on the table. It makes it too easy for everyone to overeat.

At least make people get up and get some exercise on their way for seconds!

- If you are used to "eating seconds," try this. Split your smaller portion in half, so you can look forward to having seconds but not overeating.

- If it's just you eating, don't leave the extras out if you don't want to eat them. Put the leftovers away before you sit down.

- When you buy produce (fruits, vegetables, and starches), buy the smallest pieces you can find. Look for small apples, bananas, and potatoes. Or buy large pieces and be prepared to eat only half.

- When you buy meat, fish, or poultry, buy what you need for the meal rather than too much. This can help prevent overeating. If you are making hamburgers for four and want 3-ounce cooked hamburgers, then buy 16 ounces (1 pound) of meat. If you are buying smoked turkey at the deli to make four sandwiches with 2 ounces of meat each, then buy as close to 1/2 pound (8 ounces) as you can. Make each sandwich with an equal amount of turkey.

Tips and Tricks to Control Portions of Restaurant Foods

- Steer clear of items with portion descriptors that mean "large" (unless you intend to split them). Among these terms are "giant," "grande," "supreme," "extra-large," "jumbo," "double," "triple," "double-decker," "king size," and "super."

- Seek out portion descriptors that shout "small"—"junior," "single," "petite," "kiddie," and "regular."

- Avoid all-you-can-eat restaurants and buffets. They encourage overeating.

- Don't fall for deals in which the "value" is to serve you more food so that you can save money. That's not a value to you. Opt for smaller amounts of tasty food.

- Be creative with the menu. Don't automatically order a main course. Opt for a soup and salad, an appetizer and soup, or a half portion. Or eat family style and share a few items with your dining partners. This is easy to do in Asian restaurants and is getting easier in other restaurants with the movement toward smaller plates (also called tapas).

- Split, share, and mix and match menu items to get what you want to eat in the portion you want to eat it. That's menu creativity!

- Use the fine-tuned estimating abilities that you have mastered from weighing and measuring your foods at home. Estimate what you should be eating rather than eating what they serve you. Use your eyes and those handy hand guides at the ends of your arms.

- If you know that the portion you'll be served will be too large, ask for a take-home container when you place your order. Put away the "second serving" before you dig in.

Need more help with healthy restaurant eating? Consider buying a copy of the book **Eat Out, Eat Well,** published by the American Diabetes Association (www.ShopDiabetes.org).

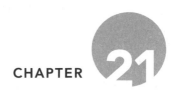

CHAPTER

Lean on the Food Label and Nutrition Facts

What's Ahead?

- ➡ How the food label and the Nutrition Facts label can help you choose healthy foods and eat proper servings.
- ➡ Information required on a food label and a Nutrition Facts label.
- ➡ Foods that must have a Nutrition Facts label.
- ➡ Similarities and differences in serving sizes between the food label and the diabetes serving sizes.
- ➡ Meaning of nutrition claims and health claims.
- ➡ Tips for using the food label and the Nutrition Facts label to make healthy food choices.

The Food Label: A Fountain of Facts

With today's food labels, you have more useful and accurate nutrition information at your fingertips than ever before. Although all of this information can be overwhelming, you can easily learn how to make sense of it and use it to help you make healthy food choices. Think of food labels as your personal nutrition assistant in the supermarket. Food labels include everything from the name of the product to the Nutrition Facts label.

Much of what you see on food labels is required by federal laws or regulations implemented by the Food and Drug Administration (FDA). The U.S. Department of Agriculture (USDA) regulates meat and poultry products. USDA regulations generally parallel the FDA's regulations. The current nutrition labeling regulations were implemented in 1994. Since then, the only major change occurred in 2006, when information about trans fat and certain food allergens became required by law. There are currently proposed regulations from the FDA to overhaul the Nutrition Facts label (such as including "added sugars" on the label, see p. 198 in chapter 14), but it will likely be a few years before there are any changes. Read more here: www.fda.gov/Food/GuidanceRegulation/GuidanceDocuments RegulatoryInformation/LabelingNutrition/ucm385663.htm. Stay up to date on these changes at FDA.gov.

What's on the Label?

You'll find the following information on food labels:

- Name of product.
- Weight of product.
- Address of manufacturer.
- Ingredients used in product, listed in descending order by weight.
- Nutrition Facts label with specific nutrition information per serving.

Sometimes you'll also find various health or nutrition claims, such as "low-fat" or "high in whole grains." These statements, defined later in this chapter, can only be made if certain criteria are met. Other times, you'll see words such as "natural" or "made with real fruit." These terms aren't regulated and are essentially marketing buzzwords used to make you think a product is healthier than it is.

Which Foods Have the Facts?

Nutrition labeling is required for almost all packaged and processed foods, but there are a few exceptions: very small packages of food with no room on the label; bulk foods like cereals or nuts that are sold from barrels; foods with no nutrients, like coffee, tea, spices, and herbs; and foods produced by very small companies.

Nutrition information for fresh fruits, vegetables, meat, poultry, and seafood, which don't have nutrition labeling, can sometimes be found posted near the product in the supermarket, on the FDA's website, on the USDA's comprehensive nutrient database (ndb.nal. usda.gov), or on many of the websites and apps listed in chapter 18. Nutrition information for foods served in restaurants is covered in chapter 22.

The Fine Print of the Nutrition Facts Label

Most Nutrition Facts labels must contain certain key information. Some products, because of their size or the type of product, can use an abbreviated label that provides less information. Some manufacturers choose to provide more information or are required to do so because of one or more nutrition or health claims they make for the food. Find the Nutrition Facts label from a frozen entrée of Enchiladas with Spanish Rice and Beans on page 280 and the explanation of each term on pages 281–282.

Serving Sizes Are Your Reference

Manufacturers can no longer make up serving sizes for their foods. The FDA has standards for serving sizes for nearly 150 categories of foods, and companies must use these standards. The standard servings are intended to be a typical serving, but they tend, for many people, to be on the small side. (In reality, they provide you with a sense of how much of a food you should actually eat!) The serving size must also be provided in household measures, such as cup or tablespoon, or it must list the number of items, so you can get a good sense of the quantity. For example, the serving size on a cracker label might read 15 crackers (28 g/1 oz). The nutrition information provided on the Nutrition Facts label is for one serving of most foods.

FDA Serving Sizes versus Serving Sizes in American Diabetes Association Resources

The standard FDA-defined serving sizes may or may not be the same as the servings sizes used in this book and other American Diabetes Association resources. You'll get to know the common serving sizes used in diabetes resources (this book, for example) and be able to compare them to the Nutrition Facts label serving sizes. Table 21.1 gives you a few examples. You'll see that some servings are the same and some are different.

If the serving sizes are the same, then it is easy to use the Nutrition Facts label as is. If they are different and you want to assess the Nutrition Facts label for one serving, you'll need to do some math. For example, suppose you're reading the label of regular salad dressing and the serving size is 2 tablespoons. The serving size in

TABLE 21.1 Comparison of Food Serving Sizes		
Food	Nutrition Label Serving	American Diabetes Association Serving
Refrigerated yogurt (fat-free, plain)	1 cup	2/3 cup
Ice cream (light or frozen yogurt)	1/2 cup	1/2 cup
Dry cereal	30 g/oz	1/2 cup
Salad dressing (reduced-fat)	2 Tbsp	2 Tbsp
Butter or margarine (regular stick)	1 Tbsp	1 tsp
Fruit juice	8 oz	1/3–1/2 cup
Salad dressing (regular)	2 Tbsp	1 Tbsp

American Diabetes Association resources is 1 tablespoon. To get nutrient information for 1 tablespoon, you need to divide the numbers on the Nutrition Facts label by 2.

Nutrition Claims Tell All

Nutrition claims on food packaging must be backed by scientific evidence. Don't just read the bold nutrition claims without checking out the numbers on the Nutrition Facts label. The food labeling law requires that manufacturers give you information to support their nutrition claims. Also, only certain nutrition claims are allowed. Some nutrition claims and their meanings are listed in Table 21.2.

TABLE 21.2 Nutrition Claim Definitions	
Nutrition Claim	**What the Nutrition Claim Means**
Free	The product contains no amount of, or only trivial amounts of, one or more of these: fat, saturated fat, cholesterol, sodium, sugars, and calories. For example, "calorie-free" means fewer than 5 calories per serving, and "sugar-free" and "fat-free" both mean less than 0.5 grams per serving. Synonyms for "free" include "without," "no," and "zero." A synonym for fat-free milk is "skim."
Low	This term can be used on foods that you can eat often without easily exceeding the dietary guidelines. "Low" can be used for fat, saturated fat, cholesterol, sodium, and calories. These are the definitions: • Low-fat: 3 grams or less per serving. • Low saturated fat: 1 gram or less per serving. • Low-sodium: 140 milligrams or less per serving. • Very low sodium: 35 milligrams or less per serving. • Low-cholesterol: 20 milligrams or less and 2 grams or less of saturated fat per serving. • Low-calorie: 40 calories or less per serving. Synonyms for "low" include "little," "few," "low source of," and "contains a small amount of."
Reduced	The product is different from the regular version and contains at least 25% less of a nutrient or of calories (e.g., reduced-fat salad dressing).

continued

TABLE 21.2 *continued*	
Nutrition Claim	**What the Nutrition Claim Means**
Less	The food, whether altered or not, contains 25% less of a nutrient or of calories than the regular food. For example, pretzels that have 25% less fat than potato chips could carry a "less" claim. "Fewer" is an acceptable synonym.
Lean and Extra Lean	This describes the fat content of meat, poultry, seafood, and game meats. • *Lean:* less than 10 grams of fat, 4.5 grams saturated fat, and 95 milligrams of cholesterol per 100-gram serving. • *Extra lean:* less than 5 grams of fat, 2 grams of saturated fat, and 95 milligrams of cholesterol per 100-gram serving.
Good and Excellent	"Good source of" means that a serving of the food provides 10–19% of the daily values for a nutrient. "Excellent source of" means that a serving of the food provides 20% or more of the daily value for a nutrient. Labels can also state "high in" or "rich in."
Healthy	Food manufacturers are allowed to use the term "healthy" if a food is low in fat and saturated fat, contains 600 milligrams or less sodium per serving for foods that are a meal entrée and 480 milligrams or less per serving for individual foods, and contains at least 10% of the daily value of vitamin A, vitamin C, calcium, iron, fiber, or protein.
More	"More" refers to a food that is 10% or more of the daily value when it is compared to a standard serving of the food without the added nutrients. Other terms that can be used instead of "more" are "enriched," "fortified," and "added."
Light	"Light" can mean two things: • A food that is nutritionally altered contains one-third fewer calories or half the fat of the regular food. If the food contains 50% or more of its calories from fat, the reduction must be 50% of the fat. • The sodium content of a low-calorie, low-fat food has been reduced by 50%. Also, "light in sodium" may be used on food in which the sodium content has been reduced by at least 50%. The term "light" still can be used to describe the texture and color of a food, as long as the label explains the intent—for example, "light brown sugar" and "light and fluffy."

Beware of Nutrition Marketing Buzzwords

In addition to the information required by law to be on food packaging, food manufacturers and marketers use a host of other terms to describe their products and, of course, to try to get you to buy them. Often, they use terms that aren't regulated or clearly defined in an attempt to make foods seem healthier than they are. Some of these buzzwords are listed in Table 21.3.

Test the Nutrition Facts Label

Use the Nutrition Facts label to see if the foods you buy or new foods you want to purchase are actually a healthy food choice. Read the food label and the Nutrition Facts label carefully, and then answer questions on pages 282–283.

TABLE 21.3	Nutrition Marketing Buzzwords
Organic	"Organic" refers to the way ingredients were grown or processed. Specific requirements must be met in order for a product to be labeled as organic. To date, there is no solid research to suggest that products labeled "organic" are healthier. They are often more expensive.
Natural	"Natural" is not regulated by the FDA, yet it's a common marketing buzzword. This term doesn't generally speak to a food's nutritional content, ingredients, safety, or healthfulness.
Made with real fruit Contains real fruit juice	There is no law that defines how much real fruit or real fruit juice must be in a product to make this claim. If you see these words, chances are there is very little real fruit used and it's likely a high-sugar product trying to masquerade as healthy. Look for products with "100% real fruit" or "100% real fruit juice" instead.
Made with whole grain 100% wheat Multigrain X grams of whole grain	Foods that use these terms are likely made with refined flour. Look for "100% whole grain" or check the ingredients list to make sure terms like "whole wheat" (not just "wheat") are first on the list.

A — # Nutrition Facts

B — **Serving Size** 1 package (285g)

C — **Servings Per Container** 1

Amount Per Serving

D — **Calories** 330   **Calories from Fat** 50

P — % Daily Value*

E — **Total Fat** 8 g	**12%**
F — Saturated Fat 1g	**5%**
Trans Fat 0g	
G — **Cholesterol** 0 mg	**0%**
H — **Sodium** 740 mg	**31%**
I — **Total Carbohydrate** 53 g	**18%**
J — Dietary Fiber 9 g	**36%**
Sugars 4 g	

K — **Protein** 9 g

L — Vitamin A 20%	•	Vitamin C 30%
Calcium 6%	•	Iron 15%

M — *Percent Daily Values are based on a 2,000 calorie diet. Your Daily Values may be higher or lower depending on your calorie needs.

	Calories:	2,000	2,500
N — Total Fat	Less than	65g	80g
Sat Fat	Less than	20g	25g
Cholesterol	Less than	300mg	300mg
Sodium	Less than	2,400mg	2,400mg
Total Carbohydrate		300g	375g
Dietary Fiber		25g	30g

O — Calories per gram:

Fat 9   •   Carbohydrate 4   •   Protein 4

A Closer Look at the Nutrition Facts Label

A **Title:** Nutrition Facts.

B **Serving Size.**

C **Servings Per Container.** The nutrition information is for one serving. For example, this frozen entrée contains one serving, so the nutrition information is for the whole package.

D **Calories** and the number of Calories from Fat in one serving.

E **Total Fat** is the total number of grams of fat in one serving.

F **The two types of fat that must be listed are Saturated Fat and Trans Fat.** Note that this information is indented from Total Fat and is in lighter print to indicate that these two types of fat are subcategories of Total Fat. Trans fat has been required on the Nutrition Facts label since 2006. Manufacturers may also choose to list monounsaturated and polyunsaturated fat; however, if a nutrition or health claim is made, they must provide this information.

G **Cholesterol** is listed in milligrams.

H **Sodium** is listed in milligrams.

I **Total Carbohydrate** is the total number of grams of carbohydrate in one serving.

J **The grams of two types of carbohydrates**—Dietary Fiber and Sugars—must be listed under Total Carbohydrate. Manufacturers may choose to list other sources of carbohydrate, such as insoluble or soluble fiber or sugar alcohols. This information is required if health or nutrition claims are made. Dietary fiber and sugars are indented and are in lighter print to indicate that they are subcategories of Total Carbohydrate.

K **Protein** is the grams of protein in one serving.

L **Vitamins and Minerals.** The percentage of the Recommended Daily Intake (RDI) in the food for vitamins A and C and two minerals, calcium and iron, must be listed. If a nutrition claim is made about another vitamin or mineral, the percentage of RDI in the food for that vitamin

continued

or mineral must be on the label. For example, if a manufacturer states, "One serving provides the daily requirement for B vitamins," the label must include nutrition information for all the B vitamins. Dry cereals often make these claims. Manufacturers can list the nutrition content for other vitamins and minerals if they want.

M **% Daily Values message.**

N **The Daily Values** are based on the amounts of each nutrient needed by a person who eats 2,000 calories a day. It's like a mini meal plan on the label. Larger packages also must list the daily values for 2,500 calories a day. Although 2,000 calories is considered an average calorie level for adults, this level is too high for many people with diabetes who need to lose weight.

O **Calories per gram:** Some of the longer labels tell you that fat has 9 calories per gram, carbohydrate has 4, and protein has 4.

P **% Daily Values** for total fat, saturated fat, cholesterol, sodium, total carbohydrate, and dietary fiber are listed to the right of each nutrient. These numbers tell you what percentage of the daily value for 2,000 calories per day is in one serving of the food. Learn more about Daily Value (DV) in chapter 5. DVs and the amount of the vitamin or mineral that a food must have per serving to use the nutrition claim: "excellent source of" or "good source of" are covered earlier in this chapter. If you eat more or fewer calories, then your personal daily values (DVs) will be different from those on the label.

- Is the portion realistic for you, or will you need to count it as more than one serving?

- How many calories are in one serving?

- How many grams of fat are in one serving? What is your daily value for fat?

- Do the advertising and nutrition claims on the front match with information from the Nutrition Facts label?

Other Items on Food Packages

Ingredients: The FDA requires that ingredients be listed in descending order by weight, so the first ingredient is the one present in the greatest amount. The last ingredient is present in the smallest amount. Use the ingredients list and the Nutrition Facts label to learn about the contents of your foods.

Food Allergens: As of 2006, the FDA requires food labels to clearly state whether they contain ingredients that cause problems for people with some food allergies. Food manufacturers are required to identify, in plain English, the presence of ingredients that contain protein derived from milk, eggs, fish, crustacean shellfish, tree nuts, peanuts, wheat, or soybeans in the list of ingredients or to say "contains" followed by name of the source of the food allergen after or next to the list of ingredients. For example, if a food contains the milk-derived protein casein, the product's label will have to use the term "milk" in addition to the term "casein," so that people with milk allergies can clearly understand that there is milk in the food. New rules for labeling gluten-free foods went into effect in 2014.

Nutrition Claim: If a nutrition claim is made on the label, the nutrition facts that justify the claim must be provided. For example, if this food carried the nutrition claim "high in monounsaturated fats," then the Nutrition Facts label would have to provide the grams of monounsaturated fat.

- Does the food fit into your eating plan and, if so, in which food group or groups?

- Are you comfortable having this food in the house, or is it better to not have it around so you avoid the temptation?

- If it is a ready-to-eat convenience food that is expensive, can you make a healthier and less expensive version at home? A homemade recipe can be lower in calories, fat, and sodium and contain fewer additives. For example, consider making your own hot cocoa, popcorn, soup, and pasta dishes.

Guides for the Supermarket Aisles

Gather shopping guidelines for different food groups below to shop for the healthiest foods.

GRAINS
- Buy your favorites and try new ones: brown rice, couscous, quinoa, barley, millet, and bulgur. Look for the most whole grains and fiber per serving.
- Buy the plain grains, not the boxed ones with seasonings that likely boost the sodium and fat content.
- You can easily store dry grains for a long time, so it's no problem to keep them on hand for a quick meal.

HOT CEREALS
- Buy whole grains: oatmeal, oat bran, or quinoa.
- Have a few on hand for variety.
- Look for cereals with the most whole grains and fiber per serving.
- Use a combination of water and fat-free milk when you prepare hot cereals for more calcium.

DRY CEREALS
- Buy whole-grain and high-fiber cereals.
- Look for 4–5 grams of dietary fiber per serving (at least).
- Keep the sugars under 5–6 grams per serving and fat below 1–2 grams.
- Think about mixing and matching a few cereals to get the nutrition mix you need but still satisfy your taste buds.

PASTA AND NOODLES
- Buy the dry kind; they are the least expensive and store the longest.

- Purchase the whole-wheat or whole-grain variety for extra fiber and other nutrients.

- Steer clear of heat-and-eat mixes with extra fat and sodium.

BREADS, BAGELS, AND ROLLS

- Go for whole-wheat or whole-grain varieties.

- Get at least 2–3 grams of dietary fiber per serving.

- Cut the fat by cutting down on biscuits, croissants, doughnuts, and higher-fat specialty breads, such as prepared garlic or focaccia bread.

CRACKERS

- Buy fat-free and reduced-fat types, but be sure they really are what they claim to be.

- Keep fat to 1–2 grams per serving.

- Buy whole-grain varieties to get 1–2 grams of dietary fiber per serving.

STARCHY SNACK FOODS

- Go for naturally fat-free and whole-grain pretzels and baked tortilla chips.

- Purchase light, fat-free, and reduced-fat varieties, but make sure they are what they say.

BEANS

- Have several types of dried beans on hand. They store well and are easy to prepare in bulk.

- Stock a few types of canned beans. If they're available in a low-sodium variety, purchase these or remember to rinse them before using. They're very quick to prepare and are versatile.

- Buy fat-free varieties of refried beans, baked beans, and vegetarian chili.

STARCHY VEGETABLES

- Have whole raw potatoes on hand to cook in the microwave.
- Try red (new) potatoes or Yukon gold potatoes. They are small, sweet, tasty types of potatoes.
- Buy fresh sweet potatoes and winter squashes; they stay fresh for a couple of weeks and are packed with vitamins and minerals.
- Keep frozen corn and green peas around. Sprinkle them on salads or in soups, or use them as a healthy starch serving.

NONSTARCHY VEGETABLES

- Eat fresh or frozen vegetables often.
- Keep canned (low-sodium) or frozen ones in your kitchen, so you'll always have vegetables on hand.
- Avoid frozen vegetables with high-fat sauces and seasonings.
- Keep individual cans of vegetable juice (regular or low-sodium, depending on your needs) on hand for a quick gulp of vegetables.

FRUITS

- Eat fresh, whole pieces of fruit often. Purchase small pieces, or plan on cutting a larger fruit into smaller portions.
- Buy canned or frozen no-sugar-added fruit or fruit packed in its own juice. Keep it in your kitchen so you'll always have fruit on hand.
- When you buy fruit juice, make sure you look for 100% fruit juice.
- Avoid fruit drinks and fruit-flavored carbonated drinks that contain a lot of calories.

MILKS AND YOGURTS

- Look for fat-free products.
- For yogurt, choose sugar-free; fat-free, sugar-free; or fat-free.
- Choose calcium-fortified fat-free milk if you can find it.

RED MEATS: BEEF, LAMB, PORK, AND VEAL

- Choose leaner cuts as often as possible.

- Go for lean or extra-lean ground meat.

- Buy lean or extra-lean cold cuts and hot dogs.

- Buy only as much as you intend to serve.

POULTRY

- The skinless breast with no wing is lowest in fat. However, consider your options and your budget, and purchase what is best for you.

- Take advantage of the availability of raw and cooked turkey breast, raw turkey legs, and cutlets.

- Buy ground turkey or low-fat turkey sausage to replace some or all of the ground meat in recipes. Check the label; ground turkey with the skin included is higher in fat.

- Usually a whole bird is cheapest, whereas boneless breast is most expensive per pound.

SEAFOOD

- Keep canned tuna (water-packed), salmon, crabmeat, clams, or imitation crabmeat on hand for a quick meal.

- Buy any type of fresh or frozen fish (not breaded).

- Choose the higher-fat fish (salmon, mackerel, or bluefish) to boost your intake of omega-3 fats.

CHEESE

- Choose cheeses with less than 5 grams of fat per ounce: light, part-skim, and reduced-calorie versions.

- Buy 1% or fat-free cottage cheese. (To control the sodium, you can buy no-salt-added or low-sodium cottage cheese.)

FATS AND OILS

- Oil: Stock one healthy all-purpose oil, such as canola or sunflower oil. (You might try a blend of soy and canola oils that is very low in saturated fat.)
- Stock extra-virgin olive oil if you enjoy the taste in salad dressings and in cooking. It's low in saturated fat.
- Margarine and spreads: Use a light tub variety (about 5 grams of fat per tablespoon). Try to get one that has zero trans fats.
- Mayonnaise: Use low-fat or reduced-calorie (about 5 grams of fat per tablespoon) mayonnaise.
- Salad dressing: Reduced-calorie dressing has about 5 grams of fat per 2 tablespoons; fat-free has less than 20–30 calories per 2 tablespoons. Or, make your own using healthy oils.
- Sour cream and cream cheese: Use light or fat-free types, as long as you enjoy the taste.

COOKIES AND CAKES

- Only buy these treats if you can control the portions you eat.
- Try to buy ones that do not contain any partially hydrogenated oils (check the ingredients list).

FROZEN DESSERTS

- Buy light and fat-free varieties, but remember that they are not calorie-free.
- Keep calories in the 100–150 range per 1/2-cup serving.

FREE FOODS

- Keep plenty of fat-free items in the pantry, such as herbs, spices, certain sauces, and seasonings. They add flavor to low-fat meals.

SOUPS

- Keep cans or dry packages on hand for quick meals or snacks. Look for the reduced- or low-sodium types.

- Buy broth-based or bean-based soups and limit the creamy varieties. Opt for lower-sodium versions.

- Dry packages work well as a snack or when you are traveling.

- Dry packages of vegetable, onion, or other soups can double as dip mix. Make sure you watch the sodium content, though.

FROZEN ENTRÉES

- Buy reduced-calorie or low-fat varieties to limit fat and keep serving sizes under control.

- Keep fat to about 3 grams per 100 grams of food.

- Keep sodium to 600–800 milligrams per entrée serving.

PIZZA

- Keep frozen cheese pizza on hand and top it with fresh vegetables.

- Choose a whole-grain pizza crust.

- Make your own. Purchase a pizza crust, pita bread, or bagel, and add your own tomato sauce, part-skim cheese, and vegetables.

CHAPTER 22

Skills and Strategies for Healthy Restaurant Eating

What's Ahead?

→ Why it's challenging to eat healthful meals at restaurants.
→ Key skills and strategies for eating healthier restaurant meals.
→ How to put healthier restaurant meals together to fit your healthy eating plan.
→ Healthier choices for a variety of popular types of restaurants.

Restaurant Meals

Restaurant eating is a way of life in America. Some Americans eat at least one meal out each day. On average, Americans eat five restaurant meals per week, and we spend about half of our food dollars on restaurant foods. About one-quarter of these meals are at or from restaurants we consider fast food, such as subs and sandwiches, burgers and fries, pizza, as well as some ethnic foods.

You can eat and enjoy restaurant meals, even with diabetes. It will, however, be important to learn how to make healthy choices with restaurant meals. This chapter will give you the key skills and strategies you need for healthy restaurant eating. For more in-depth content, pick up a copy of the book **Eat Out, Eat Well: The Guide to Healthier Restaurant Eating** published by the American Diabetes Association.

Getting to Know Yourself

If you want to change your habits with restaurant meals, the types of restaurants you eat in, and the foods you eat there, take a few minutes to do an assessment. Ask yourself the following questions to learn about your habits. Then set a few SMART goals to work to change them over time.

When do you eat out?

- Think about an average day, week, or month. Estimate the number of meals and snacks you eat away from home. Do not forget meals and snacks that you purchase at restaurants and eat somewhere else.

- Compare how often you eat out on weekdays and weekends.

Which meals and snacks do you eat away from home during an average day, week, or month?

- Breakfast, lunch, or dinner?

- Morning, afternoon, evening, or bedtime snacks?

Why do you eat restaurant meals?

- Restaurant meals are convenient.

- I do not like to cook.

- I want to have someone serve me.

- I enjoy various ethnic flavors that I cannot create in my kitchen.

- I need a place and way to get together with friends, family, or business associates.

- I want to relax during lunch or at dinner after a long day.

What types of restaurants do you choose?

- Fast food (hamburger, chicken, or seafood chains).

- Pizza or sub shops.

- American fare (family restaurant, steakhouse, or upscale continental cuisine).

- Ethnic fare (fast food or table service).

- Sweets, desserts, or ice cream.

Which foods do you eat in the restaurants listed above and in what amounts?

- Write down what you usually order in the restaurants you go to (including beverages).

- Observe the foods you eat at different types of restaurants.

- How do the servings compare with the servings in your eating plan?

- Are some food groups missing from restaurant meals that should be part of your eating plan?

Do you drink alcoholic beverages when you eat restaurant meals?

- If yes, how many alcoholic drinks do you have when you eat out?

- What alcoholic beverages do you usually drink?

- What is the calorie content of these alcoholic beverages?

Do you drink non-alcoholic beverages when you eat restaurant meals?

• If yes, how many non alcoholic drinks do you have when you eat out?

• What non alcoholic beverages do you usually drink?

• What is the calorie content of these non alcoholic beverages?

Challenges to Healthful Restaurant Eating

Here are the four main challenges to eating healthier restaurant meals. Knowing these will help you apply the key skills and strategies you'll read about next.

1. **Restaurant foods can be high in fat and high in calories.** By now you know that fat makes food taste good. Restaurants love to use oils or shortening to fry; butter and cream to create sauces; salad dressing on salads; sour cream on baked potatoes; cheese or cheese sauce on sandwiches; and butter, cream, and eggs to make desserts.

2. **Restaurant foods can be high in sodium.** The high sodium content comes from the sodium naturally in these foods and the salt that is added at the restaurant: ingredients like soy sauce, meat tenderizers, broth, ham, or bacon; sauces and gravies; items that are processed prior to entering the restaurant, like pieces of chicken; use of prepared canned food such as soups and vegetables; and salad dressings. If you need to limit sodium and you eat a lot of restaurant meals, you may have to figure out how to eat out less often. When you do eat out, limit the high-sodium foods, just as you do when you're eating at home. Asian cuisines (Japanese, Chinese, and Thai) can be quite high in sodium.

3. **Restaurant meals can be high in protein (meat, poultry, or seafood).** This is particularly true in American-style restaurants where the attention is on the main course. Steakhouses,

delicatessens, sandwich shops, and family restaurants all focus the attention on the meats.

4. **Restaurant portions can be way too large.** In America, the theory seems to be that more food equals greater value, and Americans get taken in by this message. Unfortunately, it often encourages overeating. Resisting these meal deals can be difficult.

Skills and Strategies Galore

Use these skills and strategies to rethink the way you approach restaurant meals. Use them when you eat restaurant meals.

Have a Can-Do Attitude

To manage the #1 restaurant eating challenge, treat every restaurant meal as a special occasion. If you believe that all restaurant meals are special occasions, even though you eat them several times a week, it's time for you to perform a mental mind shift— every meal can't qualify as a special occasion. If you apply the special occasion mentality that it's fine to eat larger portions, splurge on a dessert, or have a higher-fat side dish or entrée, you need to revamp your thinking. How much? That depends on your nutrition and diabetes goals.

Be honest with yourself about how you treat restaurant meals. You'll need to learn how to eat and enjoy a healthy restaurant meal without going overboard with portions or high-fat and high-sodium foods. You'll need to learn to sit back and relish other aspects of restaurant meals, like not having to clear and clean the dishes!

Select a Restaurant with Care

Today you can go into most restaurants and order a healthy meal if you choose carefully. Most menus offer at least some healthier items, or you can be creative with the menu and design a healthy meal. There are restaurants where eating a healthy meal is nearly impossible, but don't set yourself up for defeat; select restaurants that offer you at least a few healthy options.

Have a Game Plan

When you enter a restaurant, have in mind what you will order. It's likely that you've been to this restaurant many times and know the menu quite well. If you're not familiar with the restaurant, you may find the menu on the restaurant's website. Review it beforehand. Don't let the menu tempt you and steer you off track.

Be a Knowledgeable Fat Detective

You know that restaurant foods load on the fat. It is easy to keep a lid on fats if you learn these things:

- The foods that are high in fats and calories, such as butter, cream, mayonnaise, sour cream, salad dressing, cheese, sausage, nuts, and avocado.

- The cooking methods described on the menu that add fat, such as fried, deep-fried, battered and fried, golden brown, crispy, sautéed in butter, and served in a cream sauce.

- The names of high-fat dishes, such as chimichangas (Mexican), fettuccini alfredo (Italian), and sweet-and-sour whatever (Chinese).

Hold Down the Sodium

Once you can spot the high-sodium offenders, steer clear or cut down on them and make a few reasonable special requests (keep reading for more on special requests). Chapter 4, which covers salt and sodium, provides you with some tips to reduce sodium when you eat out.

Use Menu Descriptions

Menu descriptions can help you find healthier options. Look for foods such as broth-based or bean-based soups, tomato sauce, foods that come with lettuce and tomato, fat-free or low-calorie salad dressing, or fresh fruit. Some foods are naturally low in fat and calories, such as vegetables, pasta, dried beans, herbs, and spices. Look for healthier cooking methods (described on the menu), such as marinated, poached, grilled, blackened, served in a light wine sauce, or topped with sautéed garden vegetables. Look for dishes that have healthier ingredients, such as fajitas (ask for the guacamole and sour cream to be held or served on the side), yu hsiang chicken (Chinese), and pasta primavera (be careful that the sauce does not have cream added).

Be Creative with Menus

Do not feel that you have to order an entrée if the portions seem huge. If restaurants serve too much food, then order from the appetizers, soups, salads, and side dishes portions of the menu. Mix and match items to get the amount of food you need to eat.

Split Menu Items

Because servings are so large, there is often enough for two people. (You might need to order an extra side dish.) For example, one person orders an 8-ounce (raw weight) sirloin steak, a baked potato, and a trip to the salad bar. The other person orders an extra baked potato and a trip to the salad bar. Split the steak. Then it is just the right size, about 3 ounces of cooked meat for each person. You can read many more portion-control tips for restaurant eating in chapter 19.

If you are dining alone, split with yourself. Request a take-home container when you order and, when your order arrives, put half away to take home or to work for another meal.

If you enjoy splitting and sharing dishes, you'll be happy to know that in many ethnic cuisines, family-style service is customary. Entire dishes are placed in the middle of the table to share. You decide how large your serving will be. Consider ordering fewer dishes than the number of people at the table.

Share Menu Items

Share two or more menu items (depending on the number of people dining) that complement each other and achieve the goals of your healthy eating plan. This technique outsmarts the large protein servings. For example, in an Italian restaurant, one dining partner orders chicken cacciatore, which probably has about 6–8 ounces of chicken. The other partner orders pasta with a light tomato, marinara, or bolognese sauce. When you split the two dishes, each person ends up with 3–4 ounces of chicken and 1–1 1/2 cups of pasta. Order your own dinner salad for more vegetables, and order the dressing on the side.

Special Requests

Special requests can help you trim away fat and calories. Get comfortable making reasonable special requests, but don't ask or expect to have a menu item recreated in the kitchen. For example, don't try to ask for fish and chips to be turned into grilled fish with a baked potato on the side. You've just created a completely different dish! But do feel comfortable asking in a Chinese restaurant for the chicken in a dish to be sautéed rather than battered and fried. These are reasonable special requests:

- Please serve salad dressing, butter, or sour cream on the side.

- Please remove from the table or do not bring any bread and butter, chips and salsa, or Chinese noodles.

- Can the chef grill or broil this meat (poultry or seafood) rather than fry it?

- Please hold the sour cream, guacamole, shredded cheese, or olives.

- Please split this entrée into 2 servings in the kitchen, or bring us an extra plate so we can share.

- Can you serve this sandwich on whole-wheat bread rather than on a croissant?

- Can you hold the mayonnaise and bring me mustard?

- Please bring me a take-home container when you bring the meals.

Let Your Eating Plan Be Your Guide

Visualize a couple of restaurant meals. The first consists of a fast-food quarter-pound hamburger, french fries, a side salad with Thousand Island dressing, and a regular soda. The second is a Mexican meal with a basket of chips and salsa, a combo plate with one chicken taco and one beef enchilada, Mexican rice, refried beans, and a dessert of flan (Mexican custard). Both meals paint the common picture of restaurant meals: heavy on fats, meats, and sweets and light on milk, vegetables, and whole grains. Fruit is nowhere to be seen. As you know by now, these meals are not good examples of healthy eating.

Let your eating plan be your guide. Until you have your eating plan committed to memory, keep a copy in your wallet as a handy reference. Look at the menu and consider your eating plan. Here are some examples of how to apply the skills and strategies of healthy restaurant eating.

- See how you can work in whole grains. For example, are you in a Chinese restaurant that offers brown rice as an option instead of white rice? Are you eating breakfast out and do you have the option of whole-grain pancakes?

- In a sub shop, get more vegetables by asking them to load on the lettuce, tomatoes, and onions and lighten up on the fat by leaving off mayonnaise and oil.

- To fit in fruit, you'll often need to bring it with you and eat it when you are back in your car or as a snack later.

To help you further understand how to let your eating plan be your guide with restaurant meals and how to apply the skills and strategies of healthy restaurant eating, here are some sample healthy restaurant meals based on the actual nutrition information from actual restaurants. These meals show you how to closely match the number of servings from the various eating plans to some restaurant meals. Note that the sodium content of several of these meals is high, which is a challenge with restaurant eating. Refer to the end of this chapter to learn where to find nutrition information for the popular chain restaurants.

Healthier Restaurant Meals

LUNCH AT SUBWAY
(based on 1,200–1,400 calories a day)

Total Servings: 3 Starch, 1 Fruit, 2 Vegetable, 2 Protein

6-inch Roast Beef Sandwich on Honey Oat Bread (highest in fiber) (hold the oil, go light on the mayonnaise, and request plenty of lettuce, tomatoes, and onions)

Veggie Delite Salad

Italian Dressing, Fat-free

Apple Slices

> Calories: 445
> Calories from Fat: 50
> Total Fat: 6 g
> Saturated Fat: 1.5 g
> Trans Fat: 0 g
> Cholesterol: 40 mg
> Sodium: 1,463 mg
> Total Carbohydrate: 70 g
> Protein: 28 g

DINNER AT FAZOLI'S ITALIAN RESTAURANT
(based on 1,200–1,400 calories a day)

Total Servings: 3 Starch, 2 Vegetable, 1 Protein, 4 Fat
Light Baked Spaghetti, topped with broccoli
Side Chopped Salad
Dressing (request olive oil and vinegar; use 1 tsp oil and unlimited vinegar)

> Calories: 545
> Calories from Fat: 255
> Total Fat: 29 g
> Saturated Fat: 11 g
> Trans Fat: 0 g
> Cholesterol: 45 mg
> Sodium: 930 mg
> Total Carbohydrate: 50 g
> Protein: 20 g

BREAKFAST AT AU BON PAIN
(based on 1,400–1,600 calories a day)

Total Servings: 3 Starch, 1 Fruit, 1 Milk
Raisin Bran Muffin (split in half)
Banana (split in half)
Cafe Latte (16 ounce)

> Calories: 395
> Calories from Fat: 108
> Total Fat: 12 g
> Saturated Fat: 5 g
> Trans Fat: 0 g
> Cholesterol: 32 mg
> Sodium: 410 mg
> Total Carbohydrate: 62 g
> Protein: 12 g

DINNER AT CHIPOTLE'S MEXICAN RESTAURANT
(based on 1,400–1,600 calories a day)

Total Servings: 3 Starch, 1 Vegetable, 4 Protein, 1 Fat
Burrito:
  1 flour tortilla
  Carnitas (pork) (1 serving)

Fajita Vegetables (1 serving)
Roasted Chile Corn Salsa

> Calories: 530
> Calories from Fat: 216
> Total Fat: 24 g
> Saturated Fat: 8 g
> Trans Fat: 0 g
> Cholesterol: 65 mg
> Sodium: 1,310 mg
> Total Carbohydrate: 50 g
> Protein: 31 g

LUNCH AT PIZZA HUT
(based on 1,900–2,300 calories a day)

Total Servings: 5 Starch, 2 Vegetable, 3 Protein, 4 Fat
Thin 'n' Crispy Veggie Lover's Pizza (3 slices from large pizza)

> Calories: 720
> Calories from Fat: 240
> Total Fat: 27 g
> Saturated Fat: 12 g
> Trans Fat: 0 g
> Cholesterol: 60 mg
> Sodium: 2,310 mg
> Total Carbohydrate: 90 g
> Protein: 30 g

DINNER AT BOSTON MARKET
(based on 1,900–2,300 calories a day)

Total Servings: 3 Starch (corn and butternut squash are starchy vegetables),
    1 Fruit, 1 Vegetable, 5 Protein
1/4 White Meat Rotisserie Chicken (no skin)
Sweet Corn (1 serving)
Garlicky Spinach (1 serving)
Cinnamon Apples (split in half)

> Calories: 575
> Calories from Fat: 153
> Total Fat: 17 g
> Saturated Fat: 7 g

Trans Fat: 0 g
Cholesterol: 170 mg
Sodium: 1,010 mg
Total Carbohydrate: 59 g
Protein: 59 g

Healthier Restaurant Offerings by Type

Table 22.1 shows you some of the healthier and not-so-healthy offerings at various types of restaurants. As you review the lists, think about what you typically order in this type of restaurant. Then think about a few changes you could make to eat healthier offerings.

How to Find Nutrition Information for Restaurants

If you frequently eat restaurant meals, you'll want to seek out the nutritional content of the foods you eat. That's no sweat when it comes to large counter-service restaurants. It's more difficult to get the complete nutrition information from sit-down restaurants, particularly those that are small businesses or serve ethnic food. However, more and more restaurants are open about the nutrition values for the foods they serve.

Some restaurants are being forced to provide this information because of a regulation enacted in 2010 within the Patient Protection and Affordable Care Act (Obamacare) and put into effect in late 2016. This regulation amended (revised) the Food, Drug, and Cosmetic Act to require that chain restaurants, retail food establishments, and vending machines provide nutrition information for their menu items if they met certain criteria. These criteria were *1)* the business has 20 or more outlets in the U.S., *2)* the outlets were all doing business under the same name, and *3)* all outlets were offering mostly the same menu items to customers.

This regulation's focus is on calories, not on nutrients like carbohydrate or saturated fat, which are important to people with diabetes. The calories in a certain dish must be listed adjacent to the item

TABLE 22.1	Healthy and Not-So-Healthy Restaurant Choices
Healthier choices	**Not-so-healthy choices**
FAST-FOOD HAMBURGER CHAINS	
Hamburger or cheeseburger, single	Hamburger or cheeseburger,
Grilled chicken sandwich	double, triple, deluxe
Grilled chicken salad	Fried fish sandwich
Baked potato, with chili or broccoli	Fried chicken sandwich
French fries, small or share larger	Chicken nuggets or other fried
Garden and side salads	chicken pieces
Salad dressings, use light or use less	Baked potato with cheese sauce
Chef salad (light dressing)	
Roast beef sandwich	
Kid's meals with fruits and vegetables	
ROTISSERIE CHICKEN CHAINS	
White or dark meat chicken (remove	Dark meat, with skin
the skin), rotisserie, BBQ, grilled	Chicken, fried
preparation	Chicken pot pie
Ham or turkey	Caesar salad with dressing
Chicken soup	Coleslaw
Apples and cinnamon	Creamed spinach or corn
Corn bread or muffin	Macaroni and cheese
Baked beans	Pasta salad
Corn	Stuffing
Fruit salad	Meat sandwiches with cheese sauce
Green beans	Chicken salad sandwiches
Spinach	
Potatoes, mashed, pieces, baked	
Rice	
Steamed vegetables	
Zucchini in tomato sauce	
MEXICAN RESTAURANTS	
Black bean soup, tortilla soup, or	Chili con queso
gazpacho	Flautas
Mexican or taco salad without the	Nachos or super nachos
shell	Tacos (hard shell)
Arroz con pollo (chicken and rice)	Chimichangas
Burritos	*Note:* To eat less fat, ask for cheese,
Enchiladas	sour cream, or guacamole on the
Fajitas	side. Request extra salsa to add
Soft tacos	flavor.
Black beans	
Mexican rice	
Pico de gallo	
Hot sauces, all	

TABLE 22.1

Healthier choices	Not-so-healthy choices
CHINESE RESTAURANTS	
Wonton, egg drop, or hot-and-sour soup	Egg or spring roll
Steamed Peking dumpling	Jumbo shrimp
Teriyaki beef or chicken	Meat and nut dishes
Chop suey or chow mein	Deep-fried dishes
Moo shi chicken, etc.	General Tso's chicken
Shrimp with tomato sauce	Sweet-and-sour shrimp, chicken, pork, etc.
Vegetarian stir-fry dishes	Peking duck
	Spareribs
ITALIAN RESTAURANTS	
Italian bread (hold the butter)	Garlic bread or rolls
Marinated vegetable salad	Fried mozzarella cheese sticks
Minestrone soup	Caesar salad with dressing
Shrimp cocktail	Cannelloni, lasagna
Pasta with tomato sauce, marinara, bolognese, meatballs, red or white clam sauce	Pasta with pesto
	Sausage and peppers
Chicken or veal cacciatore, with light wine, or light tomato sauce	Pasta with cream and cheese sauces, alfredo, carbonara
Chicken or shrimp primavera (no cream in the sauce)	Chicken or veal parmigiana
PIZZA AND SUB SHOPS	
Cheese pizza on thin crust, loaded with vegetables	Cheese pizza on thick crust with sausage, pepperoni, or extra cheese
Submarine sandwiches with turkey, ham, roast beef, cheese (hold the oil and mayonnaise, and add vegetables)	Submarine sandwiches with tuna, chicken, or seafood salad; Italian cold cuts
AMERICAN RESTAURANTS	
Broth-based soup	New England clam chowder
Chili	French onion soup
Peel-and-eat shrimp	Buffalo wings
Salad with light or fat-free salad dressing (on the side)	Potato skins
	Tuna melt
Salad with grilled tuna or chicken	Philadelphia cheese steak
Baked potato topped with chili	Quiche
Fajitas	Ribs, beef or pork
Stir-fry chicken with vegetables	
Teriyaki chicken breast	

on the menu. In addition to calorie information, a clear and prominent statement must be posted on menus and menu boards stating that additional nutrition information for standard menu items will be made available to consumers on request.

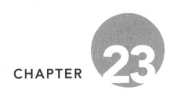

CHAPTER 23

Get the Support You Need

What's Ahead?

➡ Why it's important to always keep learning about diabetes.

➡ How to find a diabetes educator or diabetes education program.

➡ How to figure out if diabetes education and support and nutrition therapy are covered by your health plan.

➡ How to go local or global for diabetes support and engage with others with diabetes.

Healthy Eating: A Key to Diabetes Care

The positive effects of a healthy eating plan and weight loss (if need be) on your ABCs may be most significant when you are first diagnosed with prediabetes or type 2 diabetes. At these early points in the disease progression, healthy eating matched with regular physical activity can help you lose a few pounds. For some people, especially those with prediabetes, taking the steps of eating healthier, being physically active, and losing weight may be just what they needed to do to bring their ABC numbers into their target ranges and keep them there for a time.

However, many people, according to the American Diabetes Association guidelines, especially those with type 2 diabetes, need to start on at least one blood glucose–lowering medication at diagnosis. As you know from chapter 1, over time both prediabetes and type 2 diabetes often progress even if you are eating healthy, being active, and keeping those lost pounds off. It's just the reality of the disease as we know it today. This progression calls on you to be vigilant about tracking your ABCs and bringing any disease progression you detect, as well as any signs or symptoms of complications, to the attention of your health-care providers. Take this on as your job. It's your body. Keep your health-care providers on their toes by being knowledgeable about and asking for the tests and checks that are recommended for regular and annual checkups to detect early signs and symptoms of diabetes complications.

Keep in mind that even though you may need to take medication to control your blood glucose, lipids, and blood pressure, healthy eating will always help you achieve your ABC goals more easily and may even help you require less medication over time.

Get the Know-How You Need to Succeed

Learning what you need to know to get and stay healthy takes time and effort. Plus, the knowledge about managing diabetes and the tools we have to manage it are constantly evolving. This means you'll need to be constantly learning about diabetes from reputable sources. When you learn about diabetes, including from the Internet, be sure that it's from a trustworthy source, like the American Diabetes Association.

Keep reading and learning. Knowledge is power! However, knowing doesn't automatically translate to doing. Making the transition to living a healthier lifestyle is tough work that requires significant, ongoing commitment. Be kind to yourself; remember that new lifestyle changes come slowly, but they can stick as long as you take a can-do attitude. Tackle easy habits first, and reward yourself for your successes.

Get the Support You Need to Succeed

Research has proven that you will need regular and continuous support to be successful now and later on in your life with diabetes. Today, with all of the communication technology available, it's easier than ever to get the support you need from diabetes educators and diabetes education programs using apps, e-mail, online communities, video chatting, and the list goes on. Maybe you're the one looking for help, or you can be the person who offers some helpful advice to someone else with diabetes.

Where to Get Knowledge and Support

Seek out a diabetes education program offered by diabetes educators (these individuals may be CDEs, Certified Diabetes Educators). Or find a registered dietitian/nutritionist (RD or RDN) who has expertise in diabetes care. Having these providers on your side as your advocates and as resources for knowledge and support is essential to helping you strive for long-term health.

Think of these experts in diabetes care and education as your coaches and part of your all-important cheerleading squad. They can be there for you when you need a lift or an "atta boy" or "atta girl." Increasingly, these services are available through the Internet, be it through a computer or mobile device, or over the phone. Make sure that any program you use is built on strong science and supported by credentialed health professionals. Research which programs may be available to you by consulting your health-care providers, insurance provider, employer, friends, or loved ones.

Find Diabetes Education Programs or Diabetes Educators

According to the American Diabetes Association, everyone with diabetes should receive what's referred to as Diabetes Self-Management Education and Support (DSMES) initially at diagnosis and on an ongoing basis. DSMES is not simply one appointment with a diabetes educator, just attending a series of group classes, or being handed information in your health-care provider's office. DSMES encompasses initial education on the various aspects of managing diabetes day to day, from healthy eating to being more physically active to healthy coping, and it includes that all-important ongoing education and support. Although knowledge itself is important, DSMES helps you make those important behavior changes so you can transition to a healthier lifestyle.

To have DSMES covered by Medicare and some other health-care plans, you must attend a program that is accredited by either the American Diabetes Association or the American Association of Diabetes Educators. Here's how to find one of these programs:

- **The American Diabetes Association:** The American Diabetes Association approves diabetes education programs through an application and recognition process. Going to an American Diabetes Association "Recognized Education Program" ensures that you receive high-quality diabetes education. The services you are eligible to receive will depend on what your health plan covers or you decide to pay for. To find Recognized Education Programs in your area, go to http://professional.diabetes.org/erp_list.aspx or call the American Diabetes Association at 1-800-DIABETES (1-800-342-2383).

- **The American Association of Diabetes Educators (AADE):** Many diabetes educators belong to this professional organization. Diabetes educators may be nurses, nurse practitioners, dietitians, exercise physiologists, pharmacists, social workers, behavioral counselors, or psychologists. You'll find diabetes educators working at the American Diabetes Association Recognized Education Programs mentioned above. AADE also has a

Health-Plan Coverage and Reimbursement for DSMES and Medical Nutrition Therapy (MNT)

You may wonder if your health-care plan covers or reimburses for DSMES or Medical Nutrition Therapy (MNT) delivered by a credentialed health-care provider. MNT is essentially nutrition counseling provided by a Registered Dietitian/Registered Dietitian Nutritionist. When it comes to health-care plans and which of these services they cover, there's no simple answer. The answer depends on your plan and coverage and the state or federal regulations that apply to this plan. Coverage has improved greatly over the last decade. Today, many people who have health insurance can get coverage and reimbursement for both DSMES and MNT.

Contact your health plan or a local DSMES or MNT provider to see if these services are covered. If your health plan isn't willing to cover DSMES or MNT, you'll have to decide whether to reach into your pocket and pay for these services yourself. If this is the case, you'll come to realize it is money well spent. A few sessions with a knowledgeable diabetes educator is not that expensive when compared to the costs for medications, hospitalizations, or even a fancy restaurant meal.

process for accrediting diabetes education programs. To find an AADE-accredited program, visit www.diabeteseducator.org/ ProfessionalResources/accred/Programs.html.

If you have been diagnosed with prediabetes or believe you are at high risk of developing prediabetes, learn more at: doIhaveprediabetes.org. This website is part of an awareness campaign sponsored by the American Diabetes Association, CDC, and several other groups.

Another important step to take is to enroll in and complete a Diabetes Prevention Program. There are an increasing number of these programs available to you. You may find a program offered by your employer, at a local Y, by a diabetes education program, or even online. A reliable resource to find programs in your area is to access programs that have achieved recognition under the CDC National Diabetes Prevention Program. Typically these NDPP programs are year–long group programs facilitated by a trained lifestyle coarch. Find a listing at: htpps://nccd.cdc.gov/DDT_DPRP/Registry.aspx.

To Find Local Diabetes Support Groups

A local diabetes support group can be an invaluable resource. Here's how to find one:

- Call 1-800-DIABETES (1-800-342-2383). Find out the focus of the support group, the age range of its members, and when and where they meet.

- Call a local diabetes education program or a diabetes educator.

- Ask your pharmacist.

- Call the office of your or a local endocrinologist or diabetologist.

- Call a nearby hospital to see whether their diabetes program runs support groups.

To Find Further Diabetes Knowledge

The Internet has given rise to many online diabetes resources, which makes it easy to get information from national and international organizations, government agencies, and well-respected health and diabetes resources. Make sure that whatever resources you access offer trusted information.

Here are links to trustworthy national and international organizations and U.S. government agencies:

- American Diabetes Association: www.diabetes.org.

- National Institutes of Health's institute which deals with diabetes, National Diabetes and Digestive and Kidney Diseases: www.niddk.nih.gov.

- National Diabetes Education Program (NDEP): www.ndep.nih. gov.

- Centers for Disease Control and Prevention's diabetes division, known as the Division of Diabetes Translation: www.cdc.org/ diabetes.

- International Diabetes Federation: www.idf.org.

To Find Diabetes Support Around the Globe

With the rise of the Internet and social media, there's been a vast expansion of organization and independent websites, blogs, advocacy groups, and much more to support your diabetes self-care efforts and to offer you the opportunity to support others. It's worth trying to engage in these communities, if you can.

To dip a toe into these online waters, search for "diabetes online community." See what's out there. Then consider reading a few blogs. There are many, and they all have different goals and vantage points. Are you seeking the latest news on devices or technology? Are you looking for a blog that focuses on the emotional aspects of diabetes? The diabetes online community offers a growing, supportive network for people with diabetes and their caregivers so that they do not feel like they are tackling this challenging disease alone. Search for and find the support you want and need.

Beyond supporting each other in their individual journeys with diabetes, the diabetes online community is also increasingly engaged in advocating for people with diabetes within the U.S. and around the globe. Search for "diabetes advocacy," and you'll see how can engage in changing the world for all people with diabetes.

Good luck as you embark on this winding road toward your healthier eating habits and behaviors. Remember, set SMART goals and take one step at a time. If you take a step backwards, don't beat yourself up. Just move forward, focus on tomorrow, and get back on track. Pat yourself on the back for each and every success you experience. Let each and every small success give rise to more successes. By eating healthier and being physically active day after day, you improve your chances of achieving your ABC targets—blood glucose and A1C, blood pressure, and lipids. When you hit your targets year after year, you'll vastly increase your chances of staying healthy and living a long life!

Here's to you and your efforts! Good luck!

Index

*Note: Page numbers in **bold** indicate an in-depth discussion.*
Page numbers followed by t refer to tables.

Additional Praise for *Diabetes Meal Planning Made Easy*, 5th Edition

"Hope skillfully assists the reader in understanding why and how to find an eating plan that's right for the individual. Many helpful tips are suggested, including how to choose restaurant meals and how to get the support needed for healthy eating. This book is well worth reading and will help motivate, encourage, and empower individuals to eat healthfully to better manage diabetes."—**Marion J. Franz, MS, RDN, CDE**

"Nutrition can be such an overwhelming topic for most patients! This book does an incredible job of explaining all of the macronutrients and how they impact the body. in such an easy to understand way! The sample meals and tips throughout the book are great examples of what patients can realistically implement into their daily lives."—**Steven Edelman, MD**

"There is a lot of wise advise in this book. And it goes right to the heart of the matter, providing folks with diabetes and their loved ones the most critical, trustworthy, and up-to-date facts they need. Thanks to the practical and reasonable approach that is put forward in these pages, there's just no reason to feel confused or overwhelmed about eating well with diabetes anymore."—**William Polonsky, PhD, CDE**